BONE DENSITOMETRY FOR TECHNOLOGISTS

Bone Densitometry for Technologists

Sydney Lou Bonnick, MD, FACP
Lori Ann Lewis, MRT, CDT

Texas Woman's University, Denton, TX

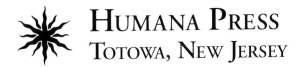

Humana Press
Totowa, New Jersey

© 2002 Humana Press Inc.
999 Riverview Drive, Suite 208
Totowa, New Jersey 07512

For additional copies, pricing for bulk purchases, and/or information about other Humana titles,
contact Humana at the above address or at any of the following numbers: Tel.: 973-256-1699;
Fax: 973-256-8341, E-mail: humana@humanapr.com; or visit our Website: http://humanapr.com

Due diligence has been taken by the publishers, editors, and authors of this book to assure the accuracy of the
information published and to describe generally accepted practices. The contributors herein have carefully
checked to ensure that the drug selections and dosages set forth in this text are accurate and in accord with the
standards accepted at the time of publication. Notwithstanding, as new research, changes in government
regulations, and knowledge from clinical experience relating to drug therapy and drug reactions constantly
occurs, the reader is advised to check the product information provided by the manufacturer of each drug for
any change in dosages or for additional warnings and contraindications. This is of utmost importance when
the recommended drug herein is a new or infrequently used drug. It is the responsibility of the treating physician
to determine dosages and treatment strategies for individual patients. Further it is the responsibility of the health
care provider to ascertain the Food and Drug Administration status of each drug or device used in their clinical
practice. The publisher, editors, and authors are not responsible for errors or omissions or for any consequences
from the application of the information presented in this book and make no warranty, express or implied, with
respect to the contents in this publication.

Cover design by Patricia F. Cleary.
This publication is printed on acid-free paper. ∞
ANSI Z39.48-1984 (American National Standards Institute) Permanence of Paper for Printed Library Ma-
terials.
Photocopy Authorization Policy:
Authorization to photocopy items for internal or personal use, or the internal or personal use of specific
clients, is granted by Humana Press Inc., provided that the base fee of US $10.00 per copy, plus US $00.25
per page, is paid directly to the Copyright Clearance Center at 222 Rosewood Drive, Danvers, MA 01923.
For those organizations that have been granted a photocopy license from the CCC, a separate system of
payment has been arranged and is acceptable to Humana Press Inc. The fee code for users of the Transactional
Reporting Service is: [1-58829-020-4/02 $10.00 + $00.25].

Printed in the United States of America. 10 9 8 7 6 5 4 3 2 1

Library of Congress Cataloging-in-Publication Data

Bonnick, Sydney Lou.
        Bone densitometry for technologists / Sydney Lou Bonnick, Lori Ann Lewis.
                p.; cm.
        Includes bibliographical references and index.
        ISBN 1-58829-020-4 (alk. paper)
        1. Bone densitometry. I. Lewis, Lori Ann. II. Title.
        [DNLM: 1. Densitometry—methods. 2. Bone Density—physiology. WE 200 B718b 2001]
        RC930.5.B678 2001
        616.7'10754—dc21   2001016675

Dedications

For Momma, Daddy and Sissy and Bo and his family
L.A.L.

For Mom and Dad, Tooney, Mabs and Charles
S.L.B.

PREFACE

Bone densitometry is an extraordinary clinical and research tool. Most of us think of densitometry as a relatively recent technological development, but in fact, its history began over 100 years ago. In the field of dentistry, crude devices by today's standards were developed in the late 19th century to evaluate the density of the bone in the mandible. The advances in technology continued, albeit slowly, for the first half of the 20th century, gaining some speed in the 1960s and 1970s. The introduction of dual energy X-ray absorptiometry in the late 1980s truly opened the door to clinicians' offices for bone densitometry. In the last 10 years the advances in technology and the introduction of new machines of various types have occurred with almost blinding speed compared to the pace of development during most of the 20th century.

As densitometry has matured as a field, the number of disease states in which bone density is known to be affected has increased. With this knowledge, physicians in many different fields of medicine now recognize the need to measure the bone density as part of the management of their patients. More studies are being requested now than ever before. This demand for densitometry has also led to an increased need for qualified technologists to operate these machines.

Densitometry is one of many quantitative techniques in use in clinical medicine today. That is, the technology is used to measure a quantity, just as the measurements of blood pressure and cholesterol are also quantitative measurement techniques. But of all the quantitative techniques in use in clinical medicine today, there is none that has the potential to be more accurate or precise than bone densitometry. The technology is highly sophisticated. All of the devices in use today employ computer technology. In spite of this mechanical sophistication, however, the technology will only be as good as the technologist.

The densitometry technologist must have knowledge of skeletal anatomy, densitometry techniques, radiation safety, basic statistics, quality control procedures, and various disease processes such as osteoporosis. The technologist must often make decisions about the conduct of testing without immediate input from the physician. The circumstances in which densitometry is usually performed create the opportunity for extended technologist–patient interaction and discussion. For technologists accustomed to performing radiologic procedures, this degree of interaction is unprecedented. Today's densitometry technologist must be prepared for these encounters.

There is no substitute for the thoughtful training provided by the manufacturers of the various types of densitometry equipment when the devices are installed. There is also no substitute for careful study of the operator's manuals that are supplied with these machines. The exact operation of each machine is different. To be proficient on any densitometry device, the technologist must be trained on that specific device. There is a broad knowledge base, however, that all technologists should possess. This text is intended to help provide that base.

It is always difficult to know where to begin. Like so many other fields of medicine, densitometry has its own language and conventions that must be explained so that in-depth discussions of densitometry are understood. Chapter 1 is an introduction to the terminology and conventions used in bone densitometry. In Chapter 2, a review of the various techniques and technologies used in quantifying the bone mass is presented (1). This review provides some of the historical development of the field as well as discussing the attributes of the various technologies and the differences between them. In Chapter 4, descriptions provided by the manufacturers of all the devices that were approved by the Food and Drug Administration at the time this book went to press can be found along with photographs of the devices. This summary description should be useful in determining what skeletal regions can be studied with any particular device, the nature of the technology employed in the device, the patient radiation exposure during a study, as well as other machine specifics. Chapter 5 covers computer basics. Although technologists and physicians are becoming more comfortable using computers and some of us consider ourselves quite "computer-literate," many of us are not. All of our machines are computer driven. A basic knowledge of computers is almost mandatory for a densitometry technologist. This chapter cannot substitute for learning the nuances of the specific software that operates any given device, but it should help those who consider themselves beginners or even intermediate computer users.

In Chapter 3, the skeletal anatomy of commonly measured densitometry sites is discussed with an emphasis on those attributes of anatomy that are either unique to densitometry or would have an effect on the measurement of bone density at that site (2). This knowledge is indispensable for the densitometry technologist. It is equally important that the technologist understand the concept of precision and how to measure it. This is presented in Chapter 6 (3). Without careful attention to precision, those factors that affect it, and knowing how to calculate it, the physician to whom the results are given will not be able to interpret followup bone density studies to determine if the bone density has changed.

All densitometers, as sophisticated as they are, are mechanical devices. Things can and do go wrong. It is imperative that machine malfunctions be recognized as soon as possible. Otherwise, the data from the machine that are provided by the technologist to the physician will be flawed. This means that a good quality control program must be in place. This is normally the responsibility of the technologist, not only to create but also to monitor. Quality control procedures are discussed in Chapter 8.

Most, but not all, densitometers are also X-ray devices. Radiation safety then must be a concern. Fortunately, both patient and technologist exposures from X-ray densitometry are incredibly small. Nevertheless, the concept of *ALARA* (as low as reasonably achievable) demands that the patient, the public, and the technologist be protected from unnecessary exposure to ionizing radiation. In Chapter 7, radiation safety concepts are discussed with recommendations made for radiation safety procedures at densitometry facilities.

The last two chapters of this book may seem unusual in a book for technologists. Chapter 9 is a review of the disease for which densitometry is most commonly used, osteoporosis. Chapter 10 is a review of how the data that come from these machines are actually interpreted. These chapters might at first seem more appropriate in a book written for physicians. The densitometry technologist, however, normally spends a significant amount of time with the patient. There is amply opportunity for the patient to ask questions of the technologist about osteoporosis and about the test that he or she is about to undergo. The knowledgeable technologist can be a vital link in the education of the patient. He or she can allay unnecessary fears and encourage appropriate medical followup. The technologist is not usurping the role of the physician by doing so if the technologist understands the issues involved. Indeed, the complete medical care of the patient must involve a partnership between the technologist and the physician. The final diagnosis and treatment recommendations for any patient must be left to the physician, but within those bounds there is much the technologist can do that will actually strengthen the patient's trust in the quality of his or her care and improve compliance with the medical recommendations. The technologist who understands as much as possible about what the physician will consider as he or she looks at the densitometry report will only be better able to aid that physician in the performance of their profession.

This technology is really quite extraordinary. The ability to quantify the density of the bones at a variety of skeletal sites has truly revolutionized the approach to a number of diseases, the most important of which is osteoporosis. Using the information from the machines, physicians can recommend and prescribe interventions that will stop bone loss and prevent disabling fractures. But it is in fact the skill and concern of the technologist that enables this to happen. It is our hope that this book assists you in your pursuit of excellence in your profession.

Sydney Lou Bonnick, MD, FACP
Lori Ann Lewis, MRT, CDT

1. Portions of this chapter were adapted from Bonnick SL (1998) Densitometry techniques in medicine today, in *Bone Densitometry in Clinical Practice*, Humana, Totowa, NJ, pp. 1–30, with permission of the publisher.
2. Portions of this chapter were adapted from Bonnick SL (1998) Densitometric anatomy, in *Bone Densitometry in Clinical Practice*, Humana, Totowa, NJ, pp. 31–64, with permission of the publisher.
3. Adapted from Bonnick SL, Johnston CC, Kleerekoper M, et al. (2001) The importance of precision in bone density measurements. *J. Clin. Densitometry. In press*. With permission of the publisher.

ACKNOWLEDGMENTS

Our gratitude is extended to the following individuals for their assistance and support in the production of this work: Joyce Paucek of Norland Medical Systems, Inc.; Christian Wulff of Osteometer Meditech; Herbert S. Lightstone of Compumed, Inc.; Nat Bowditch of Alara, Inc.; Jody Carmean, Gitte Andreasen, and Don Settergren of GE Lunar; Dave Davis and Scott Heidemann of Hologic, Inc.; Daniel Michaeli of Schick Technologies, Inc.; Dean Jenkins and Blair Rudy of Quidel Corp.; Michael Holm Hansen of Pronosco; and Imbar Vana of Sunlight Medical, Ltd.

We would also like to thank those authors and publishers who allowed us to reproduce their work in the interest of continuing education.

CONTENTS

1

An Introduction
to Conventions in Densitometry

In any discussion of bone densitometry, many terms and conventions are used that are unique to this field. In the chapters that follow, these terms and conventions are used repeatedly. In an effort to facilitate reading and comprehension, a preliminary review of some of these unique aspects of bone densitometry is offered here.

DENSITOMETRY AS A QUANTITATIVE MEASUREMENT TECHNIQUE

Bone densitometry is primarily a quantitative measurement technique. That is, the technology is used to measure a quantity, in this case, the bone mass or density. Other quantitative measurement techniques used in clinical medicine are sphygmomanometry; spirometry; and the measurement of hemoglobin, cholesterol, glucose, and other substances found in the blood. Some of today's highly sophisticated densitometers are capable of producing extraordinary skeletal images. Nevertheless, densitometry primarily remains a quantitative measurement technique, rather than an imaging technique such as plain radiography. As such, quality control measures in densitometry are not only concerned with the mechanical operation of the devices, but with attributes of quantitative measurements such as precision and accuracy.

Accuracy and Precision

Accuracy and precision are easily understood using a target analogy, as shown in Fig. 1-1. To hit the bull's-eye of the target is the goal of any archer. In a sense, the bull's-eye is the "gold standard" for accuracy. In Fig. 1-1 on target A, one of the archer's arrows has, in fact, hit the bull's-eye. Three of the other four arrows are close to the bull's-eye as well, although none has actually hit it. One arrow is above and to the right of the bull's-eye in the second ring. A second arrow is to the right and below the bull's-eye in the third ring, and a third arrow is below and to the left of the bull's-eye straddling rings two and three. The last arrow is straddling rings three and four, above and to the left of the bull's-eye. This archer can be said to be reasonably accurate, but he has been unable to reproduce his shot. Target A illustrates accuracy and lack of precision. In target B, another archer has attempted to hit the bull's-eye. Unfortunately, he has not come close. He has, however, been extremely consistent in the placement of his five arrows. All five are tightly grouped together in the upper right quadrant of the target. In other words, although not accurate, this archer's shots were extremely reproducible, or precise. Target B illustrates precision and lack of accuracy. Ideally, an archer would be both accurate and precise, as shown in target C in Fig. 1-1. Here all five arrows are grouped together within the bull's-eye, indicating a high degree of both accuracy and precision.

When bone densitometry is used to quantify the bone density for the purpose of diagnosing osteoporosis or predicting fracture risk, it is

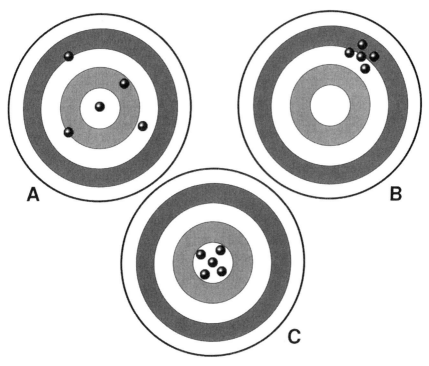

Fig. 1-1. Accuracy and precision. Target A illustrates accuracy without precision, target B illustrates precision without accuracy, and target C illustrates a high degree of both accuracy and precision.

imperative that the measurement be accurate. On the other hand, when bone densitometry is used to follow changes in bone density over time, precision becomes paramount. Strictly speaking, the initial accuracy of the measurement is no longer of major concern. It is only necessary that the measurement be reproducible or precise since it is the change between measurements that is of interest. Bone densitometry has the potential to be the most precise quantitative measurement technique in clinical medicine. The precision that is actually obtained, however, is highly dependent on the skills of the technologist. Precision itself can be quantified in a precision study, as discussed in Chapter 6. The performance of a precision study is imperative in order to provide the physician with the necessary information to interpret serial changes in bone density. Precision values are usually provided by the manufacturers for the various types of densitometry equipment. Most manufacturers express precision as a percent coefficient of variation (%CV). The %CV expresses the variability in the measurement as a percentage of the average value for a series of replicate measurements. These values are the values that the manufacturers have obtained in their own precision studies. This is not necessarily the precision that will be obtained at a clinical densitometry facility. That value must be established by the facility itself. As discussed in Chapter 6, it is preferable to use the root-mean-square standard deviation (RMS-SD) or root-mean-square coefficient of variation (RMS-CV) to express precision rather than the arithmetic mean or average standard deviation (SD) or coefficient of variation (CV). It is not always clear whether the manufacturer's precision value is being expressed as the RMS or arithmetic average. In general, the arithmetic mean SD or CV will be better than the RMS-SD or RMS-CV. Manufacturers also do not usually state the average bone density of the population in the precision study or the exact number of people and number of scans per person, making the comparison of such values with values obtained at clinical facilities difficult.

THE SKELETON IN DENSITOMETRY

Virtually every part of the skeleton can be studied with the variety of densitometers now in clinical use. The bones of the skeleton can be characterized in four different ways, one of which is unique to densitometry. The characterizations are important, because this often determines which site is the most desirable to measure in a given clinical situation. A skeletal site may be characterized as weight bearing or non–weight bearing, axial or appendicular, central or peripheral, and predominantly cortical or trabecular.

Weight Bearing or Non–Weight Bearing Sites

The distinction between weight bearing and non–weight bearing is reasonably intuitive. The lower extremities are weight bearing as is the cervical, thoracic, and lumbar spine. Often forgotten, although it is the most sensitive weight-bearing bone, is the calcaneus or os calcis. Portions of the pelvis are considered weight bearing as well. The remainder of the skeleton is considered non-weight bearing.

Axial or Appendicular Sites

The axial skeleton includes the skull, ribs, sternum, and spine, as shown in Fig. 1-2 *(1)*. In densitometry, the phrase *axial skeleton* or *axial bone*

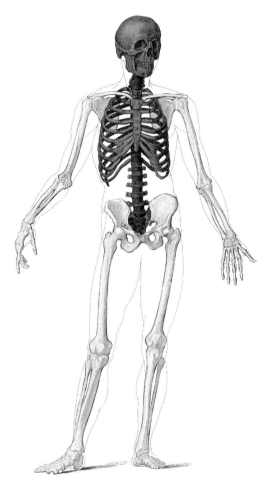

Fig. 1-2. Axial and appendicular skeleton. The darker shaded bones comprise the axial skeleton. The lighter shaded bones comprise the appendicular skeleton. Image adapted from EclectiCollections™.

density study has been used to refer to the lumbar spine and posteroanterior (PA) lumbar spine bone density studies. This limited use is no longer appropriate because the lumbar spine can also be studied in the lateral projection and the thoracic spine can be measured as well. The skull and the ribs are quantified only as part of a total body bone density study, and, as a consequence, the phrase *axial bone density study* has never implied a study of those regions. The appendicular skeleton includes the extremities and the limb girdles, as shown in Fig. 1-2. The scapulae and the pelvis are therefore part of the appendicular skeleton. The proximal femur is also obviously part of the appendicular skeleton, although it is often mistakenly included in the axial skeleton. Contributing to this confusion is the current practice of including dual energy X-ray bone density studies of the proximal femur under the CPT code 76075 used for dual X-ray (DXA) absorptiometers spine bone density studies (see Appendix V).

Central or Peripheral Sites

The characterization of skeletal sites as either central or peripheral is unique to densitometry. Central sites are the thoracic and lumbar spine in either the PA or lateral projection and the proximal femur. By extension, those densitometers that have the capability of measuring the spine and proximal femur are called central densitometers. As a matter of convention, this designation is generally not applied to quantitative computed tomography (QCT), even though spine bone density measurements are made with QCT. Peripheral sites are the commonly measured distal appendicular sites such as the calcaneus, tibia, metacarpals, phalanges, and forearm. Again, by extension, densitometers that measure only these sites are called peripheral densitometers. Some central devices also have the capability of measuring peripheral sites. Nevertheless, they retain their designation as central bone densitometers. Figure 1-3 illustrates the central and peripheral skeleton.

Cortical or Trabecular Sites

The characterization of a site as predominantly cortical or trabecular bone is important in densitometry. Some disease states show a predilection for one type of bone over the other, making this an important consideration in the selection of the site to measure when a particular disease is present or suspected. Similarly, the response to certain therapies is greater at sites that are predominantly trabecular because of the greater metabolic rate of trabecular bone. There are also circumstances in which a physician desires to assess the bone density at both a predominantly cortical and predominantly trabecular site in order to have a more complete evaluation of a patient's bone mineral status.

It is relatively easy to characterize the commonly measured sites as either predominantly cortical or predominantly trabecular, as shown in Table 1-1. It is more difficult to define exact percentages of cortical and trabecular bone at each site. The values given in Tables 1-2 and 1-3 should be considered clinically useful approximations of these percentages.

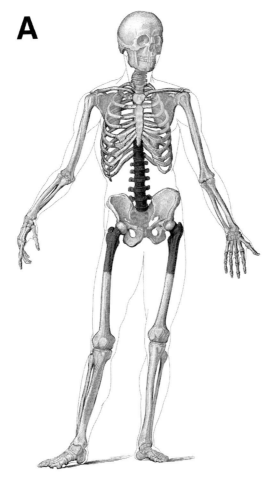

Fig. 1-3. Central and peripheral skeleton. (**A**) The darker shaded bones comprise the central skeleton. *(continued)*

Slightly different values may appear in other texts depending on the references used, but the differences tend to be so small that they are not clinically important.

Any given skeletal site can thus be characterized in four different ways. For example, the calcaneus is a weight-bearing, appendicular, peripheral, predominantly trabecular site. The femoral neck is a weight-bearing, appendicular, central, predominantly cortical site. The lumbar spine, in either the PA or lateral projection, is a weight-bearing, axial, central, predominantly trabecular site.

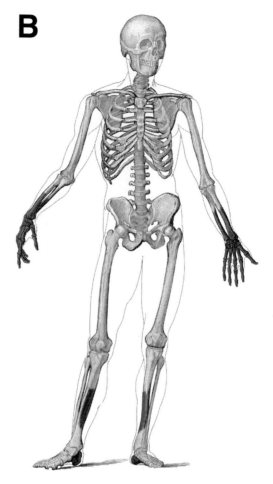

Fig. 1-3. *(continued)* **(B)** The darker shaded bones comprise the peripheral skeleton. Images adapted from EclectiCollections™.

WHAT DO THE MACHINES ACTUALLY MEASURE?

Although all of today's X-ray densitometers ultimately report bone mineral density (BMD), none actually measure BMD. Instead, the quantities that are actually measured are the bone mineral content (BMC) and the length or area of bone. BMC is usually expressed in grams although it is measured in milligrams (mg) when quantified by QCT or pQCT (peripheral quantitative computed tomography). Length is generally measured in centimeters (cm) and area in square centimeters (cm²). In the

Table 1-1
Predominantly Trabecular or Cortical Sites

Trabecular	Cortical
PA spine	Total body
Lateral spine	Femoral neck
Ward's	33% Forearm[a]
4 to 5% Forearm[a]	10% Forearm[a]
Calcaneus	5- and 8-mm Forearm[b]
	Phalanges

[a]% indicates the location of the region of interest on the radius, ulna, or both combined as a percentage of the length of the ulna, measured from the ulnar styloid. See Chapter 3 for a discussion of naming conventions for forearm sites.

[b]Distance in millimeters (mm) indicates the separation distance between the radius and ulna at the site in question. See Chapter 3 for a discussion of naming conventions for forearm sites.

Table 1-2
Percentage of Trabecular Bone at Central Sites as Measured by DXA

Site	Trabecular bone (%)
PA spine[a]	66
Lateral spine[b]	?
Femoral neck	25
Trochanter	50
Ward's[b]	?
Total body	20

[a]These percentages are only for DXA PA spine studies. A volumetric measurement of 100% trabecular bone could be obtained with QCT.

[b]These sites are considered to be highly trabecular, but the exact percentage of trabecular bone is not known.

case of QCT and pQCT, volume, not area, is measured and reported in cubic centimeters (cm^3). The BMD is calculated from the measurement of BMC and area or BMC and volume as shown in eqs. 1 and 2:

$$BMC\ (g)/Area\ (cm^2) = BMD\ (g/cm^2) \qquad (1)$$

$$BMC\ (mg)/Volume\ (cm^3) = BMD\ (mg/cm^3) \qquad (2)$$

When bone density measurements are made in the lumbar spine in the PA projection by DXA, the BMD for three or four contiguous vertebrae is generally reported rather than the BMD for any single vertebra. In other words, the L1–L4 or L2–L4 BMD is reported for the lumbar spine rather

Table 1-3

Percentage of Trabecular Bone at Peripheral Sites as Measured by SXA or DXA

Site	Trabecular bone (%)
Calcaneus	95
33% Radius or ulna[a,b]	1
10% Radius or ulna[a,c]	20
8-mm Radius or ulna[a,c]	25
5-mm Radius or ulna[a,c]	40
4 to 5% Radius or ulna[a,d]	66
Phalanges	40

[a]See Chapter 3 for naming convention for forearm bone density sites.
[b]This site is often called the *proximal* site.
[c]This site is often called the *distal* site.
[d]This site is often called the *ultradistal site* but may be called simply *distal* as well.

than only using L1, L2, L3, or L4. The accuracy and precision for L1–L4 or L2–L4 are superior to the accuracy and precision for single vertebrae. But how is the L1–L4 or L2–L4 BMD derived? The BMD is calculated by the densitometry software for each individual vertebra and these values are provided on the bone density report as shown in Fig. 1-4. It is tempting to assume that the individual BMDs for each of the vertebrae included in the three or four vertebrae value are simply added and then the total divided by the number of vertebrae to find the "average" BMD. This is not correct, however. Remember that BMD is not measured directly; it is calculated from the measurement of BMC and area. The correct approach is to add the BMC values for each of the vertebrae included in the 3 or 4 vertebrae value and divide this total by the sum of the individual areas of each of the included vertebrae. This is illustrated in eq. 3 for the L1–L4 BMD:

$$BMD_{L1-L4} = \frac{(BMC_{L1} + BMC_{L2} + BMC_{L3} + BMC_{L4})}{(Area_{L1} + Area_{L2} + Area_{L3} + Area_{L4})} \tag{3}$$

It is an accepted convention in densitometry to call the L1–L4 BMD and the L2–L4 BMD "average" BMD values, even though they do not truly represent the average of the BMD at each vertebral level.

Quantitative ultrasound (QUS) measurements of bone density do not measure BMC or area. Instead, two parameters of the passage of sound through bone are measured: speed of sound (SOS) and broadband ultrasound attenuation (BUA). The SOS is derived by determining the speed with which the sound wave passes through the bone. This requires a

TEXAS WOMAN'S UNIVERSITY
Denton, Texas

AP SPINE BONE DENSITY

Facility: TWU   Acquired: 09/15/2000 (4.7a)
47 years   Analyzed: 09/15/2000 (4.7a)
64 in 125 lbs White Female   Printed: 09/15/2000 (4.7a)
Physician: Bonnick

Region	BMD g/cm²	Young Adult %	T	Age Matched %	Z
L1	1.039	92	-0.8	94	-0.6
L2	1.081	90	-1.0	92	-0.8
L3	1.080	90	-1.0	92	-0.8
L4	1.048	87	-1.3	89	-1.1
L1-L2	1.062	92	-0.7	94	-0.5
L1-L3	1.069	91	-0.8	93	-0.7
L1-L4	1.063	90	-1.0	92	-0.8
L2-L3	1.080	90	-1.0	92	-0.8
L2-L4	1.069	89	-1.1	91	-0.9
L3-L4	1.063	89	-1.1	90	-1.0

Fig. 1-4. DXA PA spine bone density report showing the calculated BMD values for each lumbar vertebra and every combination of contiguous vertebrae. Percentage comparisons and standard scores are also shown. This is the detailed data for the summary report in Fig. 1-5.

measurement of time and distance from which the SOS is then calculated and usually expressed in meters/second (m/sec). BUA refers to the amount of energy lost from the sound wave as it passes through bone. It is expressed in decibels/megahertz (db/Mhz). Figure 1-6 shows an ultrasound bone density report. Some manufacturers will mathematically combine the SOS and BUA into a proprietary index such as the Stiffness Index, shown in Fig. 1-6.

THE DENSITOMETRY PRINTOUT

A complete printout for a PA lumbar spine study is shown in Figs. 1-4 and 1-5. In addition to reporting the measured and calculated parameters, comparisons are made by the densitometry software, using the databases contained within the computer. The purpose of these comparisons is to place the measured and calculated values into some context. Are these values good or bad? Do they indicate the presence of disease or not? Two types of comparisons are made. The first is in the form of a percentage of the average peak value for a young adult and the average value for an

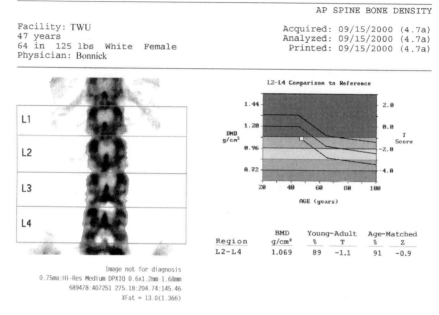

TEXAS WOMAN'S UNIVERSITY
Denton, Texas

AP SPINE BONE DENSITY

Facility: TWU
47 years
64 in 125 lbs White Female
Physician: Bonnick

Acquired: 09/15/2000 (4.7a)
Analyzed: 09/15/2000 (4.7a)
Printed: 09/15/2000 (4.7a)

Region	BMD g/cm²	Young-Adult % T	Age-Matched % Z
L2-L4	1.069	89 -1.1	91 -0.9

Image not for diagnosis
0.75ma:Hi-Res Medium DPXIQ 0.6x1.2mm 1.68mm
689478:407251 275.18:204.74:145.46
%Fat = 13.0(1.366)

Fig. 1-5. Summary DXA PA spine bone density report showing the skeletal image, age-regression graph, and data for the selected region of interest, L2–L4. Detailed data are shown for this study in Fig. 1-4.

individual the same age as the patient. The second comparison again compares the value to the expected peak value for a young adult and the expected average value for an individual the same age, but the comparisons are in the form of standard scores called T-scores and z-scores.

The Percentage Comparisons

The expression of the patient's value as a percentage of the average peak value for a young adult of the same sex is called the "% Young Adult" or the "% Young Reference" comparison. This percentage may also be found in parentheses next to the T-score. The age or age range at which peak bone density is assumed to have occurred is sometimes not clear. The age used by the manufacturers may vary for any given skeletal site and certainly varies among different skeletal sites. The age or age range for peak bone density used for the % Young Adult comparison

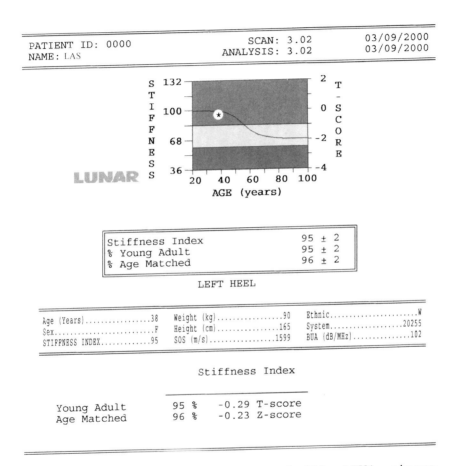

Texas Woman's University
Center for Research on Women's Health
Denton, Texas

PATIENT ID: 0000   SCAN: 3.02   03/09/2000
NAME: LAS   ANALYSIS: 3.02   03/09/2000

Stiffness Index	95 ± 2
% Young Adult	95 ± 2
% Age Matched	96 ± 2

LEFT HEEL

Age (Years)...............38   Weight (kg)................90   Ethnic......................W
Sex......................F   Height (cm)...............165   System..................20255
STIFFNESS INDEX...........95   SOS (m/s)................1599   BUA (dB/MHz)..............102

Stiffness Index

| Young Adult | 95 % | -0.29 T-score |
| Age Matched | 96 % | -0.23 Z-score |

Fig. 1-6. Ultrasound bone density report. The values for SOS and BUA can be seen in the middle section of the report. SOS and BUA have been mathematically combined to produce a proprietary index by this manufacturer, called the Stiffness Index. The value for this index is plotted on the age-regression graph. The background of the age-regression graph is divided into green, yellow, and red areas. The dividing lines for these areas correspond to the World Health Organization (WHO) diagnostic categories based on the T-score. This can be helpful but should be interpreted cautiously in younger individuals.

can be determined by reviewing information on the database that has been provided by the manufacturer or by studying the age-regression graph.

If the "% Young Adult" value for an L2–L4 PA spine BMD is 89% as shown in Fig. 1-5, the patient's BMD is 89%, of the average peak bone density for a young adult of the same sex. The BMD is 11% below the average peak bone density. This % Young-Adult value should not be interpreted as meaning that the patient has lost 11% of her bone density. After all, the patient's actual peak bone density as a young adult is not known. The patient's peak bone density could have been higher or lower than the average peak bone density. How much the patient's bone density has actually changed, if at all, cannot be determined from a single bone density study. One can only conclude that her bone density is 11% lower than the average peak.

The second comparison that is made in the form of a percentage is to compare the patient's value to the average value for an individual the same age and sex. This is usually called the "% Age-Matched" comparison, or it may be listed in parentheses next to the z-score. This percentage indicates how the patient compares with other people their same age. Unfortunately, this value can be misinterpreted, resulting in a false sense of security. Individuals tend to lose bone density with age. Although this is an expected phenomenon, it is not a desirable one. To have a bone density that compares favorably with that of other individuals of the same age who may also have lost bone density is not necessarily good. Ideally, an individual's bone density will be better than expected for their age. If the "% Age-Matched" comparison is quite poor, it raises the specter of some underlying cause of bone loss other than age or, for women, estrogen deficiency. The effects of both age and estrogen deficiency are already reflected in the values that are established as expected in the database. When the "% Age Matched" comparison is poor, something other than age or estrogen deficiency should be suspected. Nothing may necessarily be found, but other causes of bone loss should certainly be considered. It is difficult to say exactly what constitutes a "poor" comparison, but certainly anything less than 80% should raise a red flag and prompt a very thorough evaluation for other causes of bone loss.

The Standard Score Comparisons

Standard scores are not unique to densitometry, but they are not used routinely in any other field of clinical medicine. As a consequence, densitometry is usually a technologist's and physician's first exposure to standard scores. Standard scores take their name from their dependence on

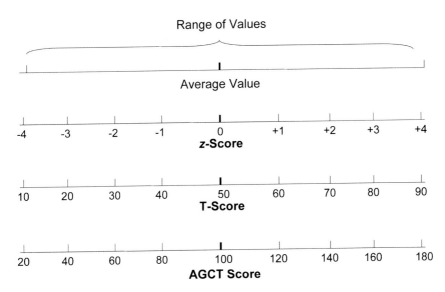

Fig. 1-7. Standard score scales. These scales are based on the SD.

the "standard" deviation (SD), a statistical measure of variability about an average value. The calculation of the SD and its utility in expressing the variability of measurements about an average value is discussed more thoroughly in Chapter 6 in the context of precision.

Standard scores indicate how many SDs above or below the average value the value in question actually lies. Several different standard score scales have been created *(2);* these scales are illustrated in Fig. 1-7. At the center of each scale is the average (also called mean) value for whatever set of values is being considered. Remember that standard scores and scales are not unique to densitometry. These scales can be applied to any kind of numerical values.

In the *z*-score scale, the *z*-score value increases by 1 for each SD increase or decrease from the average value. The average value is arbitrarily assigned a *z*-score value of 0. A plus (+) sign or minus (−) sign is placed in front of the *z*-score value to indicate whether the value lies above or below the average value. If the actual value were 2 SDs above the average, the *z*-score would be +2. If the value were 1.5 SDs below the average, the *z*-score would be −1.5.

In the T-score scale, as it was originally designed, the average value was arbitrarily assigned a T-score value of 50. For each SD change in the actual value from the average, the T-score would increase or decrease by 10. If the actual value were 1 SD above the average, the T-score would be 60. If it were 2 SDs below the average it would be 30. Another type of standard score scale is the Army General Classification Test (AGCT) scale, in which the average value is assigned an AGCT score of 100 and each SD increase or decrease from the average changes the AGCT score by 20.

Both the original T-score and AGCT scales utilize whole numbers and neither requires the use of a plus or minus sign. The z-score scale, on the other hand, does require the use of small numbers, decimal points, and either a plus or minus sign. It is perhaps unfortunate, but at present, the z-score scale is the basis for the standard score comparisons used in densitometry.

In densitometry, if a patient's z-score is −2, the implication is that the patient's value is 2 SDs below the average value. But to what average value is the comparison being made? There is nothing in the definition of the z-score that specifies the average to which the comparison is being made. Is it the average peak value of the young adult or the average value that is expected for the patient's age? In years past, this dilemma was addressed by labeling the comparisons "Young-Adult Z" and "Age-Matched Z" in order to make clear what comparison was being made. This is no longer done today. By convention in densitometry, it is understood that the z-score comparison is the comparison to the average value expected for the patient's age. The z-score scale is still used for comparisons of the patient's value to the average peak value for a young adult, but this comparison, by convention, is now called the T-score. This is clearly a misuse of the term *T-score* since it is the z-score scale that is being used, but it has served to shorten the terminology required to distinguish between the 2 comparisons without using a different standard score scale. In the bone density report shown in Fig. 1-5, the patient's L2–L4 T-score is −1.1 and her z-score is −0.9. Her L2–L4 BMD, then, is 1.1 SDs below the peak value for a young adult and 0.9 SDs below the value predicted for her age.

Like the "% Young Adult" comparison, the T-score should not be used to suggest a certain magnitude of bone loss. It is the T-score, however, on which current diagnostic criteria are based. Like the "% Age-Matched" comparison, the z-score only indicates how the patient compares with her age-matched peers. A poor z-score should prompt a thorough evaluation for causes of bone loss other than age and estrogen deficiency. Statistically, a poor z-score is anything below or poorer than −2, but certainly such an evaluation should be pursued at any time the physician deems necessary.

Because both peak bone density and the expected bone density for any age can be affected by the race and weight of an individual, the percentage comparisons and standard scores can be adjusted to take these factors into account. The various manufacturers approach this issue differently, however. In some cases, the % Young-Adult and T-score comparisons can be adjusted for race, whereas in other cases it is the % Age-Matched and z-score that are adjusted. The weight adjustment may be made similarly in either set of comparisons. A careful reading of the device manufacturer's description of the comparisons is the only way to know with certainty where these adjustments are being made.

The Age-Regression Graph

The age-regression graph on densitometry reports, while usually quite colorful, is only a graphic representation of the selected calculated parameter and the standard score comparisons for a particular region of interest (ROI). Consequently, it actually provides little to no additional information beyond the printed numbers. On these graphs, the patient's BMD (or ultrasound value) will be plotted above their age. This is superimposed on a line graph of the expected change in BMD with advancing age, called the *age-regression line*. The highest point on this graph will represent the peak BMD (or ultrasound parameter) for the young adult. On both sides and paralleling the age-regression line is an outer limiting line that denotes a 1 or 2 SD change in BMD from the predicted value for any age. Some manufacturers have used a 1 SD limit for this line whereas others have used a 2 SD limit. The limits shown on the age-regression graph in Fig. 1-5 represent a 1 SD change. These limits allow a visual estimation of the z-score. In the background of the graph, many manufacturers are now utilizing a red, yellow, and green color scheme, as shown in the QUS bone density report in Fig. 1-6. If the BMD or other chosen parameter lies in the red area, the World Health Organization (WHO) criteria for a diagnosis of osteoporosis have been met. If the plotted value is in the yellow area, the diagnosis is osteopenia, and if in the green area, the diagnosis is normal. Red, yellow, and green are also used to denote high, medium, and low risk of fracture, respectively. The WHO criteria for the diagnosis of osteoporosis are discussed more thoroughly in Chapter 9 and are listed again in Appendix II for easy reference. Although the red, yellow, and green color scheme can be useful, these colored areas extend across the entire age range represented on the graph. The WHO criteria were intended to be applied only to postmenopausal women. In addition, fracture risk at younger ages, is clearly not the same as fracture risk at older ages, even at the same BMD. As a consequence, this aspect of the graph must be interpreted with caution.

The Standardized BMD

The bone density values at any one skeletal site when obtained on devices from different manufacturers will not be the same. This is not because one device is more accurate than another; all the various devices are highly accurate as long as good quality control is maintained. The differences occur because the devices are calibrated to slightly different standards and because of slight differences in how the edges of the bones are detected. It has been shown repeatedly that the results for a skeletal site on one manufacturer's device are highly correlated with the results for that site from another manufacturer's device. In other words, the devices are indeed measuring the same thing. While the absolute values that are reported are different, they are predictably different. A useful analogy would be a certain amount of money expressed as either US dollars, Canadian dollars or British pounds. The numbers will be different even though the actual amount of money is the same.

Because the values are different, however, there has been a great deal of interest in developing a standardized BMD (sBMD) to which all DXA values could be converted regardless of which manufacturer's machine was used. In November 1990, the major manufacturers of DXA equipment agreed to work together in the area of standards as part of an international committee, known as the International Committee for Standards in Bone Measurement. Under the auspices of this committee, a study of 100 healthy women was performed in which each of the women underwent PA spine and proximal femur studies on the Hologic QDR-2000, the Norland XR-26 Mark II, and the Lunar DPX-L (3). The women ranged in age from 20 to 80 years, with an average age of 52.6 years. The difference in BMD in the spine was greatest between the Norland XR-26 and the Lunar DPX-L, averaging 0.118 g/cm^2, or 12.2%, with Lunar values being higher than Norland values. The difference between the Lunar DPX-L and the Hologic QDR-2000 averaged 0.113 g/cm^2, or 11.7%, with Lunar values again being higher. Between the Norland XR-26 and the Hologic QDR-2000, the average difference in BMD in the lumbar spine was only 0.012 g/cm^2, or 1.3%.

Based on this data, equations were derived for the conversion of PA lumbar spine BMD obtained on one manufacturer's machine to the BMD that would be expected on each of the other two. These equations for

Table 1-4
Conversion Formulas for BMDs of PA Spine Among DXA Devices

Hologic QDR-2000 $Spine_{BMD}$ = (0.906 × Lunar DPX-L $Spine_{BMD}$) − 0.025
Hologic QDR-2000 $Spine_{BMD}$ = (0.912 × Norland XR 26 $Spine_{BMD}$) + 0.088
Lunar DPX-L $Spine_{BMD}$ = (1.074 × Hologic QDR 2000 $Spine_{BMD}$) + 0.054
Lunar DPX-L $Spine_{BMD}$ = (0.995 × Norland XR 26 $Spine_{BMD}$) + 0.135
Norland XR-26 $Spine_{BMD}$ = (0.983 × Lunar DPX-L $Spine_{BMD}$) − 0.112
Norland XR-26 $Spine_{BMD}$ = (1.068 × Hologic QDR 2000 $Spine_{BMD}$) − 0.070

Adapted from *Journal of Bone and Mineral Research* 1994;9:1503–1514 with permission from the American Society for Bone and Mineral Research.

Table 1-5
Formulas for Conversion of Manufacturer-Specific AP Spine BMDs
to the Standardized BMD (sBMD)

$sBMD_{SPINE}$ = 1000(1.076 × Norland XR-26 BMD_{SPINE})
$sBMD_{SPINE}$ = 1000(0.9522 × Lunar DPX-L BMD_{SPINE})
$sBMD_{SPINE}$ = 1000(1.0755 × Hologic QDR-2000 BMD_{SPINE})

Adapted from *Journal of Bone and Mineral Research* 1994;9:1503–1514 with permission from the American Society for Bone and Mineral Research.

each of the three pairs of scanners are given in Table 1-4 and again in Appendix VII, for easy reference.

To convert each manufacturer's absolute BMD to an sBMD, a specially designed phantom called the European Spine Phantom (ESP) was scanned on each of the three devices.* Based on those results, formulas for converting each manufacturer's absolute BMD in the spine to a standardized spine BMD were derived; Table 1-5 gives these formulas.

The value for the sBMD is multiplied by 1000 to convert it to milligrams/square centimeter rather than reporting it in grams/square centimeter to distinguish the sBMD from the nonstandardized value. For example, if the L2–L4 BMD obtained in the PA spine on a Lunar DXA device is 1.069 g/cm², as shown in Fig. 1-5, this value becomes 1018 mg/cm² when reported as the sBMD (1.069 × 0.9522 = 1.0179 g/cm² × 1000 = 1018 mg/cm²). When these formulas were used to convert the average PA lumbar spine BMD for the 100 women in the study population to the

*See Chapter 8 for a discussion of the European Spine Phantom.

Table 1-6
Conversion Formulas for BMDs in Proximal Femur Among DXA Devices

Hologic QDR-2000 Neck$_{BMD}$ = (0.836 × Lunar DPX-L Neck$_{BMD}$) − 0.008
Hologic QDR-2000 Neck$_{BMD}$ = (0.836 × Norland XR 26 Neck$_{BMD}$) + 0.051
Lunar DPX-L Neck$_{BMD}$ = (1.013 × Hologic QDR 2000 Neck$_{BMD}$) + 0.142
Lunar DPX-L Neck$_{BMD}$ = (0.945 × Norland XR 26 Neck$_{BMD}$) + 0.115
Norland XR-26 Neck$_{BMD}$ = (0.961 × Lunar DPX-L Neck$_{BMD}$) − 0.037
Norland XR-26 Neck$_{BMD}$ = (1.030 × Hologic QDR 2000 Neck$_{BMD}$) + 0.058

Adapted from *Journal of Bone and Mineral Research* 1994;9:1503–1514 with permission from the American Society for Bone and Mineral Research.

Table 1-7
Formulas for Conversion of Manufacturer-Specific Total Femur BMD
to the Standardized BMD (sBMD)

sBMD$_{TOTAL FEMUR}$ = 1000 [(1.008 × Hologic BMD$_{TOTAL FEMUR}$) + 0.006]
sBMD$_{TOTAL FEMUR}$ = 1000[(0.979 × Lunar BMD$_{TOTAL FEMUR}$) − 0.031]
sBMD$_{TOTAL FEMUR}$ = 1000[(1.012 × Norland BMD$_{TOTAL FEMUR}$) + 0.026]

Adapted from *Journal of Bone and Mineral Research* 1997;12:1316, 1317 with permission from the American Society for Bone and Mineral Research.

sBMD, the differences in BMD among the three machines were greatly reduced. Instead of an average difference of 12.2% between the Norland and Lunar values, the difference using the sBMD was only 2.8%. The difference between Hologic and Lunar was reduced to 2.2%, and the difference between Hologic and Norland was 2.7%.

Conversion formulas were also developed for the femoral neck for each pair of scanners; Table 1-6 gives these formulas.

In December 1996, the International Committee for Standards in Bone Measurement approved the sBMD for the total femur region of interest *(4)*. The total femur region of interest includes the femoral neck, Ward's area, trochanter, and shaft of the proximal femur. This region appears to have equal diagnostic utility but better precision than the femoral neck. The formulas for the sBMD for the total femur, shown in Table 1-7, were based on the work by Genant et al. *(3)* from which the formulas for sBMD of the spine were also derived. The sBMD from any one of the three central DXA devices should fall within 3–6% of the sBMD on any of the other two. The sBMD calculation is generally provided as an option in most densitometry software that can be turned on and off by the technologist.

The NHANES III Database for the Proximal Femur

Although the development of the sBMD reduced the apparent discrepancies between the reported values for BMD at the PA spine and total femur among the three major DXA device manufacturers, discrepancies still remained between the percentage comparisons and standard scores. These discrepancies were seen at both the lumbar spine and the proximal femur, but the problem was clearly greatest at the proximal femur.

In 1992 Pocock et al. *(5)* noted that the percentage comparisons for the spine were similar in 46 women studied on the Hologic QDR-1000 and the Lunar DPX. At the femoral neck, however, the % Young Adult comparisons were 6.2% lower on the QDR-1000 compared with the Lunar DPX. The % Age-Matched comparisons were 3.3% lower on the QDR-1000 than on the Lunar DPX.

Other authors confirmed these observations. Laskey et al. *(6)* evaluated 53 subjects undergoing spine and proximal femur bone density measurements on the same day on the Lunar DPX and Hologic QDR-1000. Like Pocock et al. *(5)*, they found that the young-adult and age-matched comparisons to the reference database at the spine were similar. At the proximal femur, however, the differences were substantial. The magnitude of the differences approximated 1 SD. This was a sufficient difference to potentially have profound clinical ramifications. Depending on which manufacturer's machine was used for the measurement, a patient potentially could be given a different diagnosis. Faulkner et al. *(7)* compared the young adult standard scores at the spine in 83 women and at the proximal femur for 120 women who underwent bone density studies on a Lunar DPX and Hologic QDR-1000/W. The difference between the young adult standard scores on the QDR-1000/W and the Lunar DPX at the spine was not statistically or clinically significant. At the femoral neck, however, there was a systematic difference of almost 1 SD.

Faulkner et al. *(7)* observed that these differences in percentage comparisons and standard scores could be due to a combination of factors: different inclusion criteria for the two databases, relatively small numbers of individuals used to calculate the average and SD young adult values, and different statistical methods employed in the calculation of the reference curves. Faulkner suggested correcting the proximal femur data from both manufacturers by replacing the manufacturer's data with proximal femur bone density data obtained during the National Health and Nutrition Examination Survey (NHANES) III study of the US population.* These data were collected between 1988 and 1991 using the Hologic QDR-1000 *(8)*. As originally reported, there were 194 non-Hispanic white women age 20–29 whose BMD values were used to calculate the young adult average BMD value and SD in the five regions in the proximal femur. The average BMD in the femoral neck for these young adults from NHANES III was reported as 0.849 g/cm^2, with a SD of 0.11 g/cm^2. Faulkner et al. *(7)* substituted these values for the average and SD values used in the QDR-1000 reference database of 0.895 and 0.10 g/cm^2, respectively. The equivalent Lunar DPX BMD young adult BMD was then calculated using the cross-calibration equation from Genant et al. *(3)*. This resulted in a Lunar value of 1.000 g/cm^2 for the average young adult BMD in the femoral neck compared with the value of 0.980 g/cm^2 used in the Lunar-supplied database prior to October 1997. The SD for the young adult of 0.11 g/cm^2 from NHANES III was substituted for the Lunar reported SD of 0.12 g/cm^2. When the young adult standard scores were recalculated for each machine using the new values based on the NHANES III data, the differences between the two manufacturer's databases largely disappeared.

With the development of the cross-calibration equations between manufacturers and the sBMD for the total femur, it became possible for the proximal femur data from NHANES III to be adopted as a common femur database by the different manufacturers even though the original data were obtained solely on Hologic DXA devices. Based on the equations for sBMD, the average sBMD for US non-Hispanic white women age 20–29 is 956 mg/cm^2 with a SD of 123 mg/cm^2 *(4)*. Standardized NHANES III proximal femur data were offered as part of the reference databases by DXA manufacturers, either in conjunction with the manufacturer-derived databases or as a replacement for the manufacturer-derived proximal femur data after September 1997.

---

*NHANES III was conducted by the National Center for Health Statistics, Centers for Disease Control and Prevention. During the study, proximal femur bone density data were collected on 7116 men and women age 20 and older *(8)*. There was a total of 3217 non-Hispanic whites, 1831 non-Hispanic blacks, and 1840 Mexican-Americans in this study population. There were no specific inclusion or exclusion criteria used to select individuals for bone density measurements other than the presence of prior hip fracture or pregnancy, which were grounds for exclusion. The individuals who received bone density measurements were otherwise part of a random sample of the population.

REFERENCES

1. Recker, R. R. (1992) Embryology, anatomy, and microstructure of bone, in *Disorders of Bone and Mineral Metabolism* (Coe, F.L. and Favus, M.J., eds.), Raven, New York, pp. 219–240.
2. Phillips, J. L. (1982) Interpreting individual measures, in *Statistical Thinking*, W.H. Freeman, New York, pp. 62–78.
3. Genant, H. K., Grampp, S., Gluer, C. C., Faulkner, K. G., Jergas, M., Engelke, K., Hagiwara, S., Van Kuijk, C. (1994) Universal standardization for dual X-ray absorptiometry: patient and phantom cross-calibration results. *J. Bone Miner. Res.* **9**, 1503–1514.
4. Hanson, J. (1997) Standardization of femur BMD. *J. Bone Miner. Res.* **12**, 1316, 1317.
5. Pocock, N. A., Sambrook, P. N., Nguyen, T., Kelly, P., Freund, J., Eisman, J. A. (1992) Assessment of spinal and femoral bone density by dual X-ray absorptiometry: comparison of Lunar and Hologic instruments. *J. Bone Miner. Res.* **7**, 1081–1084.
6. Laskey, M. A., Crisp, A. J., Cole, T. J., Compston, J. E. (1992) Comparison of the effect of different reference data on Lunar DPX and Hologic QDR-1000 dual-energy X-ray absorptiometers. *Br. J. Radiol.* **65**, 1124–1129.
7. Faulkner, K. G., Roberts, L. A., McClung, M. R. (1996) Discrepancies in normative data between Lunar and Hologic DXA systems. *Osteoporos. Int.* **6**, 432–436.
8. Looker, A. C., Wahner, H. W., Dunn, W. L., Calvo, M. S., Harris, T. B., Heyse, S. P., Johnston, C. C., Lindsay, R. L. (1995) Proximal femur bone mineral levels of US adults. *Osteoporos. Int.* **5**, 389–409.

2 Densitometry Techniques

The field of bone densitometry has grown rapidly in the last 15 years. With the techniques now available, bone density can be quantified in almost every region of the skeleton. The clinical application of these technologies is relatively new but densitometry is actually quite old. It was first described more than 100 years ago in the field of dental radiology as dentists attempted to quantify bone density in the mandible *(1,2)*.

PLAIN RADIOGRAPHY IN
THE ASSESSMENT OF BONE DENSITY

The earliest attempts to quantify bone density utilized plain skeletal radiography. When viewed by the unaided eye, plain skeletal radiographs can only be used in an extremely limited fashion to quantify bone density. Demineralization becomes visually apparent only after 40% or more of the bone density has been lost *(3)*. If demineralization is suspected from a plain film, a great deal of demineralization is presumed to have occurred. A more precise statement cannot be made. Plain radiographs have been used for qualitative and quantitative skeletal morphometry. Plain radiographs were also used to assess bone density based on the optical densities of the skeleton when compared to simultaneously X-rayed standards of known density. With the advent of the photon absorptiometric techniques, most of these early methods as originally performed have fallen into disuse. Nevertheless, a brief review of these techniques should both enhance the appreciation of the capabilities of modern testing and provide a background for understanding modern technologies.

QUALITATIVE MORPHOMETRY

Qualitative Spinal Morphometry

Qualitative morphometric techniques for the assessment of bone density have been in limited use for more than 50 years. Grading systems for the spine relied on the appearance of the trabecular patterns within the vertebral body and the appearance and thickness of the cortical shell *(4)*. Vertebrae were graded from IV down to I as the vertical trabecular pattern became more pronounced with the loss of the horizontal trabeculae and the cortical shell became progressively thinned. The spine shown in Fig. 2-1 demonstrates a pronounced vertical trabecular pattern. The cortical shell appears as though it was outlined in white around the more radiotranslucent vertebral body. These vertebrae would be classified as Grade II.

The Singh Index

The Singh Index is a qualitative morphometric technique that was similarly based on trabecular patterns, but based on those seen in the proximal femur *(5)*. Singh and others had noted that there was a predictable

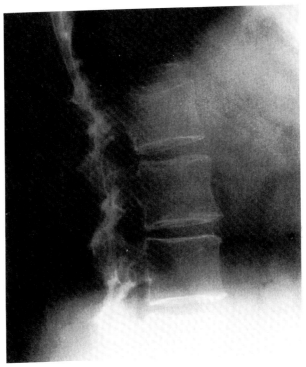

Fig. 2-1. Quantitative spine morphometry. The vertebrae on this lateral lumbar spine X-ray demonstrate marked accentuation of the vertical trabecular pattern and thinning of the cortical shell. This is a Grade II spine.

order in the disappearance of the five groups of trabeculae from the proximal femur in osteoporosis. Based on the order of disappearance, radiographs of the proximal femur could be graded 1 through 6 with lower values indicating a greater loss of the trabecular patterns normally seen in the proximal femur. Studies evaluating prevalent fractures demonstrated an association between Singh Index values of 3 or less and the presence of fractures of the hip, spine, or wrist. Figure 2-2 shows a proximal femur with a Singh Index of 2. Only the trabecular pattern known as the principle compressive group, which extends from the medial cortex of the shaft to the upper portion of the head of the femur, remains. This patient was known to have osteoporotic spine fractures as well as a contralateral proximal femur fracture. Later attempts to demonstrate an association between Singh Index values and proximal femur bone density measured by dual-photon absorptiometry were not successful (6). These

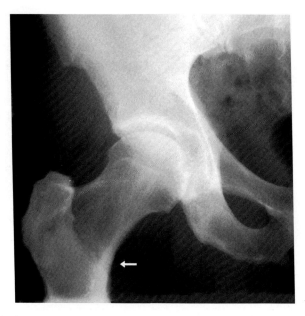

Fig. 2-2. Singh Index and calcar femorale thickness. A Grade 2 Singh Index would be assessed based on having only remnants of the principle compressive principle tensile trabecular groups visible. This is indicative of osteoporosis. The arrow points to the calcar femorale, which was 4 mm thick. Values <5 mm are associated with hip fracture. This patient had experienced a contralateral hip fracture.

qualitative morphometric techniques are highly subjective. In general, the best approach required the creation of a set of reference radiographs of the various grades to which all other radiographs could be compared.

QUANTITATIVE MORPHOMETRIC TECHNIQUES

Calcar Femorale Thickness

A little-known quantitative morphometric technique involves the measurement of the thickness of the calcar femorale. The calcar femorale is the band of cortical bone immediately above the lesser trochanter in the proximal femur. In normal subjects, the thickness is greater than 5 mm. In femoral fracture cases, it is generally less than 5 mm *(7)*. The arrow in Fig. 2-2 is pointing to the calcar femorale. This patient had previously suffered a femoral neck fracture. The thickness of the calcar femorale measured 4 mm.

Radiogrammetry

Radiogrammetry is the measurement of the dimensions of the bones using skeletal radiographs. Metacarpal radiogrammetry has been in use for almost 50 years. The dimensions of the metacarpals were measured using a plain radiograph of the hand and fine calipers or a transparent ruler. The total and medullary widths of the metacarpals of the index, long, and ring fingers were measured at the midpoint of the metacarpal. The cortical width was calculated by subtracting the medullary width from the total width. Alternatively, the cortical width could be measured directly. A variety of different calculations were then made such as the metacarpal index (MI) and the hand score (HS). The MI is the cortical width divided by the total width. The HS, which is also known as the percentage cortical thickness, is the MI expressed as a percentage. Measurements on the middle three metacarpals of both hands were also made and used to calculate the six metacarpal hand score (6HS). Other quantities derived from these measurements included the percentage cortical area, the cortical area, and the cortical area to surface area ratio. The main limitation in all of these measurements is that they were based on the false assumption that the point at which these measurements were made on the metacarpal was a perfect hollow cylinder. Nevertheless, by using these measurements and knowing the gravimetric density of bone, the bone density could be calculated. The correlation between such measurements and the weight of ashed bone was good, ranging from 0.79 to 0.85 *(8,9).** The precision of metacarpal radiogrammetry was quite variable depending on the measurement used.[†] The measurement of total width is very reproducible. The measurement of medullary width or the direct measurement of cortical width is less reproducible, because the delineation between the cortical bone and medullary canal is not as distinct as the delineation between the cortical bone and soft tissue. Precision was variously reported as excellent to poor, but in expert hands it was possible to achieve a precision of 1.9% *(10).*

---

*Correlation indicates the strength of the association between two values or variables. The correlation value is denoted with the letter *r*. A perfect correlation would be indicated by an *r* value of +1.00 or −1.00.

[†]Techniques are compared on the basis of accuracy and precision, which can be described using the percent coefficient of variation (%CV). The %CV is the standard deviation (SD) divided by the average of replicate measurements expressed as a percentage. The lower the %CV, the better the accuracy or precision. See Chapters 1 and 6 for a detailed discussion of precision and accuracy.

Although metacarpal radiogrammetry is an old technique and somewhat tedious to perform, it remains a viable means of assessing bone density in the metacarpals. Metacarpal radiogrammetry demonstrates a reasonably good correlation to bone density at other skeletal sites measured with photon absorptiometric techniques *(11)*. The technique is very safe because the biologically significant radiation dose from a hand X ray is extremely low at only 1 mrem.

Radiogrammetry can also be performed at other sites such as the phalanx, distal radius, and femur *(12–14)*. Combined measurements of the cortical widths of the distal radius and the second metacarpal have been shown to be highly correlated with bone density in the spine as measured by dual photon absorptiometry *(12)*.

Today, plain films can be digitized using flatbed optical scanners and radiogrammetry performed with computerized analysis of the digitized images. A commercially available system, the Pronosco X-posure System™, is discussed in Chapter 4.

The Radiologic Osteoporosis Score

The radiologic osteoporosis score combined aspects of both quantitative and qualitative morphometry *(14)*. Developed by Barnett and Nordin *(14)* this scoring system utilized radiogrammetry of the femoral shaft and metacarpal as well as an index of biconcavity of the lumbar vertebrae. In calculating what Barnett and Nordin *(14)* called a peripheral score, the cortical thickness of the femoral shaft divided by the diameter of the shaft and expressed as a percentage was added to a similar measurement of the metacarpal. A score of 88 or less was considered to indicate peripheral osteoporosis. The biconcavity index was calculated by dividing the middle height of usually the third lumbar vertebra by its anterior height and expressing this value as a percentage. A biconcavity index of 80 or less indicated spinal osteoporosis. Combining both the peripheral score and biconcavity index resulted in the total radiologic osteoporosis score that was considered to indicate osteoporosis if the value was 168 or less.

RADIOGRAPHIC PHOTODENSITOMETRY

Much of the development of the modern techniques of single photon absorptiometry (SPA) DPA, and dual-energy X-ray absorptiometry actually came from early work on the X-ray-based method of photodensitometry *(15)*. In photodensitometry, broad-beam X-ray exposures of radio-

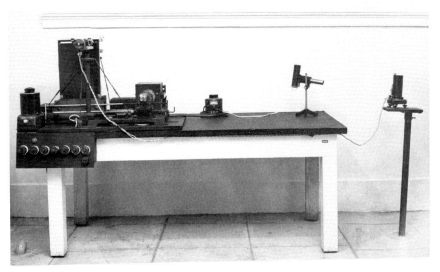

Fig. 2-3. Radiographic photodensitometer at Texas Woman's University from the early 1950s.

graphs were obtained, and the density of the skeletal image was quantified using a scanning photodensitometer. One such early device at Texas Woman's University is shown in Fig. 2-3. The effects of variations in technique such as exposure settings, beam energy, and film development were partially compensated by the simultaneous exposure of a step wedge of known densities on the film. An aluminum wedge was most often used, but other materials such as ivory were also employed *(13)*. This technique could be applied only to areas of the skeleton in which the soft-tissue coverage was less than 5 cm, such as the hand, forearm, and heel, because of technical limitations due to scattered radiation in thicker parts of the body and "beam hardening" or the preferential attenuation of the softer energies of the polychromatic X-ray beam as it passed through the body. It was also used in cadaver studies of the proximal femur *(16)*. Such studies noted the predictive power for hip fracture of the density of the region in the proximal femur known as Ward's triangle 30 years before studies using the modern technique of dual-energy X-ray absorptiometry in 1993 *(17)*.* The accuracy of such measurements was fairly good with

---

*Ward's triangle was first described by F. O. Ward in *Outlines of Human Osteology*, Henry Renshaw, London, 1838. It is a triangular region created by the intersection of three groups of trabeculae in the femoral neck.

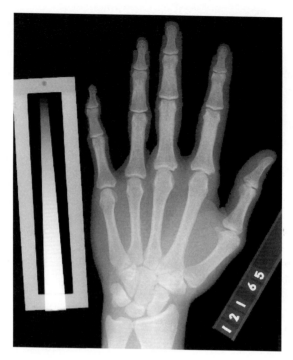

Fig. 2-4. Radiographic photodensitometry hand film taken in 1965 of one of the *Gemini* astronauts. The Texas Woman's University aluminum wedge is seen next to the little finger.

a %CV of 5%. The correlation between metacarpal photodensitometry and ashed bone was high at 0.88 *(8)*. This was a slightly better correlation than seen with metacarpal radiogrammetry. The precision of photodensitometry was not as good however ranging from 5 to 15% *(18)*. By comparison, the six metacarpal radiogrammetry hand score was superior *(4)*. Radiation dose to the hand was the same for metacarpal radiogrammetry and radiographic photodensitometry. In both cases, the biologically significant radiation dose was negligible.

Radiographic photodensitometry was developed and used extensively by researchers Pauline Beery Mack and George Vose *(19)*. Many of the original studies of the effects of weightlessness on the skeleton in the *Gemini* and *Apollo* astronauts were performed by Pauline Beery Mack and colleagues at Texas Woman's University *(20)*. Figure 2-4 shows photodensitometry hand film of one of the *Gemini* astronauts.

RADIOGRAPHIC ABSORPTIOMETRY

Radiographic absorptiometry (RA) is the modern-day descendent of radiographic photodensitometry *(21,22)*. The ability to digitize high-resolution radiographic images and to perform computerized analysis of such images has largely eliminated the errors introduced by differences in radiographic exposure techniques and overlying soft-tissue thickness. As originally performed in the United States, two X-rays of the left hand using nonscreened film were taken at slightly different exposures. Standard X-ray equipment was used to perform the hand films. The initial recommended settings were 50 kVp at 300 mA for 1 second and 60 kVp at 300 mA for 1 second. The exact settings varied slightly with the equipment used and were adjusted so that the background optical density of each of the two hand films matched a quality control film. An aluminum alloy reference wedge was placed on the film prior to exposure, parallel to the middle phalanx of the index finger. After development, the films were sent to a central laboratory where they were digitized and analyzed by computer. The average bone mineral density (BMD) in arbitrary RA units of the middle phalanxes of the index, long, and ring fingers was reported. Figure 2-5 illustrates the X-ray appearance of the hand and aluminum alloy reference wedge.

In cadaveric studies, Yang et al. *(23)* found the accuracy of RA for the assessment of bone mineral content (BMC) of the middle phalanges to be good at 4.8%. They did note that very thick soft tissue that might be seen in very obese subjects could potentially result in an underestimation of RA values. The correlation between the RA values and the ashed weight in the phalanges was excellent with $r = 0.983$. The short-term reproducibility of these measurements was also excellent at 0.6%.

The ability to predict bone density at other skeletal sites from hand RA is as good as that seen with other techniques such as single-photon absorptiometry, dual-photon absorptiometry, dual-energy X-ray absorptiometry, or quantitative computed tomography of the spine *(21,24)*. This does not mean that RA hand values can be used to accurately predict bone density at other skeletal sites. Although the correlations among the different sites as measured by the various techniques are correctly said to be statistically significant, the correlations are too weak to allow clinically useful predictions of bone mass or density at one site from measurement at another.

The utility of modern-day radiographic absorptiometry in predicting hip fracture risk was suggested by an analysis of data acquired during

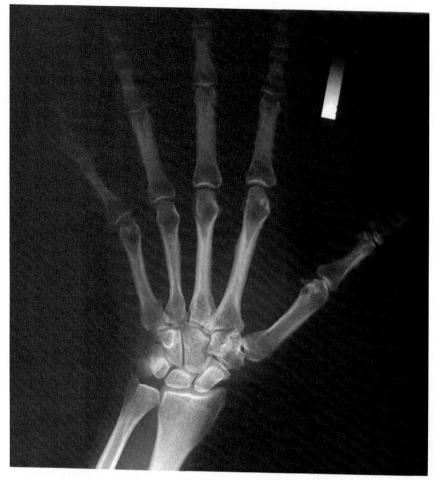

Fig. 2-5. Radiographic absorptiometry hand film. The small aluminum wedge, originally known as the Fel's wedge, is seen next to the index finger.

the first National Health and Nutrition Examination Survey (NHANES I, 1971–1975). During this survey, 1559 hand radiographs of Caucasian women were obtained with the older technique of photodensitometry using the Texas Woman's University wedge *(25)*. During a median follow-up of 14 years that extended through 1987, 51 hip fractures occurred. Based on radiographic photodensitometry of the second phalanx of the small finger of the left hand, the risk for hip fracture per standard deviation decline in bone density increased 1.66-fold. These films were then reanalyzed using RA with some compensation for the differences in technique.

This reanalysis yielded an increase in the risk for hip fracture per standard deviation decline in RA bone density of 1.81-fold. Huang et al. *(26)* evaluated the utility of RA in the prediction of vertebral fractures. They followed 560 postmenopausal women, average age 73.7 years, for an average of 2.7 years in the Hawaii Osteoporosis Study *(26)*. The risk for vertebral fracture in this study using RA was 3.41-fold for each SD decline in bone density.

RA systems are commercially available. The automated Osteogram® system from Compumed consists of the computer hardware, software, and film cassette with hand template and reference wedge needed to perform RA of the phalanges. The Metriscan™ from Alara is a self-contained device that utilizes storage phosphor technology in place of X-ray film to perform RA of the phalanges. Both systems are discussed in Chapter 4.

PHOTON ABSORPTIOMETRY TECHNIQUES

In radiology, attenuation refers to a reduction in the number and energy of photons in an X-ray beam. Attenuation, then, is a reduction in an X-ray beam's intensity. To a large extent, the attenuation of X rays is determined by tissue density. The difference in tissue densities is responsible for creating the images seen on an X ray. The more dense the tissue, the more electrons it contains. The number of electrons in the tissue determines the ability of the tissue to either attenuate or transmit the photons in the X-ray beam. The differences in the pattern of transmitted or attenuated photons creates the contrast necessary to discern images on the X ray. If all the photons were attenuated (or none were transmitted), no image would be seen because the film would be totally white. If all the photons were transmitted (or none were attenuated), no image would be seen because the film would be totally black. The difference in the attenuation of the X-ray photon energy by different tissues is responsible for the contrast on an X ray, which enables the images to be seen. If the degree of attenuation could be quantified, it would be possible to quantitatively assess the tissue density as well. This is the premise behind the measurement of bone density with photon absorptiometric techniques. The earliest photon absorptiometric techniques employed radionuclides to generate photon energy. These radionuclide-based techniques have now given way to X-ray-based techniques. The basic principles on which they operate, however, remain the same.

Single Photon Absorptiometry

In 1963, Cameron and Sorenson *(27)* described a new method for determining bone density in vivo by passing a monochromatic or single-energy photon beam through bone and soft tissue. The amount of mineral encountered by the beam could be quantified by subtracting the beam intensity after passage through the region of interest (ROI) from the initial beam intensity. In the earliest single-photon absorptiometry units, the results of multiple scan passes at a single location, usually the midradius, were averaged *(28)*. In later units, scan passes at equally spaced intervals along the bone were utilized such that the mass of mineral per unit of bone length could be calculated. A scintillation detector was used to quantify the photon energy after attenuation by the bone and soft tissue in the scan path. After the photon attenuation was quantified, a comparison with the photon attenuation seen with a calibration standard derived from dried, defatted human ashed bone of known weight was made in order to determine the amount of bone mineral.

The photon beam and the detector were highly "collimated," or restricted in size and shape. The beam source and detector moved in tandem across the region of interest on the bone, coupled by a mechanical drive system. Iodine-125 at 27.3 keV or americium-241 at 59.6 keV were originally used to generate the single energy photon beam, although most SPA units subsequently developed in the United States employed only [125]I.

The physical calculations for SPA determinations of bone mineral were valid only when there was uniform thickness of the bone and soft tissue in the scan path. To artificially create this kind of uniform thickness, the limb to be studied had to be submerged in a water bath or surrounded by a tissue-equivalent material. As a practical matter, this limited SPA to measurements of the distal appendicular skeleton such as the radius and, later, the calcaneus. Figure 2-6 is a photograph of an old SPA device, the Norland 2780, that was in use in the 1980s.

SPA was both accurate and precise although the parameters varied slightly with the site studied. For SPA measurements of the midradius, accuracy ranged from 3 to 5%, and precision from 1 to 2% *(27,29–31)*. Early measurements of the distal and ultradistal radius with SPA did not demonstrate the same high degree of precision primarily due to the marked changes in the composition of the bone with very small changes in location within the distal and ultradistal radius.* With later instruments employing

---

*See Chapter 3 for a discussion of the composition of the radius and ulna.

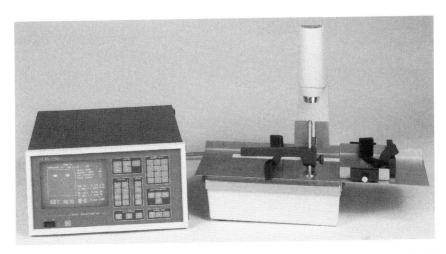

Fig. 2-6. Early Norland model 2780 single photon absorptiometer. This device utilized ^{125}I to generate photon energy. (Photo courtesy of Norland Medical Systems, Ft. Atkinson, WI.)

computer-enhanced localization routines and rectilinear scanning, SPA measurements of the distal and ultradistal radius approached a precision of 1% *(32)*. Accuracy and precision of measurements at the calcaneus with SPA were reported to be less than 3% *(30)*. The skin radiation dose for both the radius and calcaneus was 5–10 mrem *(30,31)*. The biologically important radiation dose, the effective dose, was negligible. Results were reported as either bone mineral content (BMC) in grams or as bone mineral content per unit length (BMC/l) in grams/centimeter. The time required to perform such studies was approximately 10 minutes *(33)*.

SPA is rarely performed today, having been supplanted first by single X-ray absorptiometry (SXA) and now dual-energy X-ray absorptiometry. The demise of SPA was because of improvements in ease of use and precision seen with SXA and DXA. SPA was an accurate technology that could be used to predict fracture risk. The ability to predict the risk of appendicular fractures with SPA measurements of the radius was convincingly established *(34–36)*. SPA measurements of the radius were also good predictors of spine fracture risk and global fracture risk *(34,37,38)*.* Indeed, the longest fracture trials published to date, demonstrating the

---

*Global fracture risk refers to the risk of having any and all types of fractures combined. This is in contrast to a site-specific fracture risk prediction in which the risk for a fracture at a specific skeletal site is given, such as spine fracture risk or hip fracture risk.

ability of a single bone mass measurement to predict fracture, were performed using SPA measurements of the radius.

Dual Photon Absorptiometry

The basic principle involved in dual-photon absorptiometry (DPA) for the measurement of bone density was the same as for SPA: quantifying the degree of attenuation of a photon energy beam after passage through bone and soft tissue. In dual photon systems, however, an isotope that emitted photon energy at two distinct photoelectric peaks or two isotopes, each emitting photon energy at separate and distinct photoelectric peaks, were used. When the beam was passed through a region of the body containing both bone and soft tissue, attenuation of the photon beam occurred at both energy peaks. If one energy peak was preferentially attenuated by bone, however, the contributions of soft tissue in beam attenuation could be mathematically subtracted (39). As in SPA, the remaining contributions of beam attenuation from bone were quantified and then compared to standards created from ashed bone. The ability to separate bone from soft tissue in this manner finally allowed quantification of the bone density in those areas of the skeleton that were surrounded by large or irregular soft-tissue masses, notably the spine and proximal femur, DPA was also used to determine total body bone density. The development of DPA and its application to the spine, proximal femur, and total body is attributed to a number of investigators: B.O. Roos, G.W. Reed, R.B. Mazess, C.R. Wilson, M. Madsen, W. Peppler, B.L. Riggs, W.L. Dunn and H.W. Wahner (40–45).

The isotope most commonly employed in DPA in the United States was gadolinium-153, which naturally emitted photon energy at two photoelectric peaks, 44 and 100 keV. At the photoelectric peak of 44 keV, bone preferentially attenuated the photon energy. The attenuated photon beams were detected by a NaI scintillation detector and quantified after passage through pulse-height analyzers set at 44 and 100 keV. The shielded holder for the ^{153}Gd source, which was collimated and equipped with a shutter that was operated by a computer, moved in tandem with the NaI detector in a rectilinear scan path over the region of interest. A point-by-point calculation of bone density in the scan path was made. Figure 2-7 is an intensity-modulated image of the spine created with an early DPA device.

DPA bone density studies of the lumbar spine were performed with the photon energy beam passing in a posterior to anterior direction. Because of the direction of the beam, the vertebral body and the posterior elements were included in the scan path. The transverse processes were eliminated.

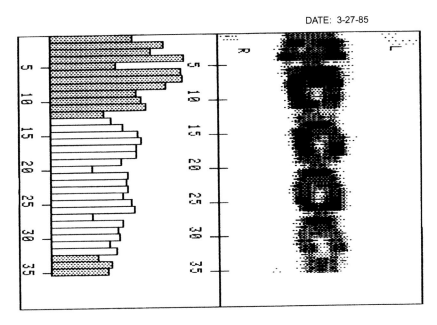

DATE: 3-27-85

Fig. 2-7. A dual photon posteroanterior (PA) spine study obtained on a device as shown in Fig. 2-8. The spine image is upside down. The histogram at the left was used to place the intervertebral disc space markers. The shortest bar in the vicinity of the disc space was identified and the marker was placed there.

This resulted in a combined measurement of cortical and trabecular bone, or integral measurement, that included the more trabecular vertebral body surrounded by its cortical shell and the highly cortical posterior elements. The results were reported as an areal density in grams/square centimeter. The BMD of the proximal femur was also an areal density that was acquired with the beam passing in a posterior to anterior direction. Figure 2-8 shows an early dual photon absorptiometer with the patient positioned for a study of the lumbar spine.

DPA studies of the spine required approximately 30 minutes to complete, studies of the proximal femur took 30–45 minutes, and total body bone density studies with DPA required 1 hour. Skin radiation dose was low during spine or proximal femur studies at 15 mrem. Accuracy of DPA measurements of the spine ranged from 3 to 6% and for the proximal femur 3 to 4% *(46)*. Precision for measurements of spine bone density was 2–4% and about 4% for the femoral neck.

DPA was considered a major advance from SPA because it allowed the quantification of bone density in the spine and proximal femur. DPA

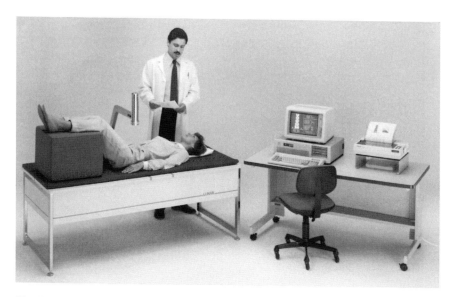

Fig. 2-8. Early GE Lunar DP3 dual photon absorptiometer. This device utilized [153]Gd to generate photon energy. (Photo courtesy of GE Lunar, Madison, WI.)

did have several limitations, however. Machine maintenance was expensive. The [153]Gd source had to be replaced yearly at a cost of $5000 or more. It had also been noted that as the radioactive source decayed, values obtained with DPA increased by as much as 0.6% per month *(47)*. With replacement of the source, values could fall by as much as 6.2%. Although mathematical formulas were developed to compensate for the effect of source decay, it remained a cause for concern, potentially affecting both accuracy and precision. The precision of 2 to 4% for DPA measurements of the spine and proximal femur limited its application in detecting changes in bone density. With a precision of 2%, a change of at least 5.5% from the baseline value had to be seen before one could be certain at the 95% confidence level that any change had occurred at all *(48)*. With a precision of 4%, this figure increased to 11.1%. At a lower 80% confidence level, the required changed for precision values of 2 and 4% were 3.6 and 7.2%, respectively. As a practical matter, this meant that DPA bone density studies would not show significant changes for 2 to 5 years at a minimum. This was too long a period to wait to be clinically useful.

In DPA spine bone density studies in which the photon beam passed in a PA direction, the highly trabecular vertebral body could not be separated from its more cortical posterior elements. In addition, the cortical shell of the vertebral body could not be separated from its trabecular interior. Calcifications in the overlying soft tissue or abdominal aorta will attenuate such a beam, falsely elevating the bone density values. Arthritic changes in the posterior elements of the spine also affect the measurement *(49)*. These effects are discussed in greater detail in Chapter 3. PA dual energy X-ray absorptiometry (DXA) studies of the spine are not immune to these effects either, but lateral DXA spine studies can be performed to overcome these limitations. Studies of the spine in the lateral projection were never available with DPA.

The ability to make site-specific predictions of fracture risk of the spine and proximal femur or global fracture risk predictions with DPA was established in prospective trials *(17,37)*. Like SPA, DPA is rarely performed in the United States now, because of the availability of DXA with its technological improvements.

Dual-Energy X-Ray Absorptiometry

The underlying principles of dual-energy X-ray absorptiometry (DXA) are the same as those of DPA. With DXA, however, the radioactive isotope source of photon energy has been replaced by an X-ray tube. There are several advantages of X-ray sources over radioactive isotopes. There is no source decay that would otherwise require costly replacement of the radioactive source. Similarly, there is no concern of a drift in patient values from source decay. In addition, the greater source intensity or "photon flux" produced by the X-ray tube and the smaller focal spot allows for better beam collimation, resulting in less dose overlap between scan lines and greater image resolution. Scan times are faster and precision is improved.

Because X-ray tubes produce a beam that spans a wide range of photon energies, the beam must be narrowed in some fashion in order to produce the two distinct photoelectric peaks necessary to separate bone from soft tissue. The major manufacturers of central dual X-ray absorptiometers in the United States have chosen to do this in one of two ways. GE Lunar (Madison, WI) and Norland Medical Systems (Fort Atkinson, WI) use rare-earth K-edge filters to produce two distinct photoelectric peaks. Hologic (Bedford, MA) uses a pulsed power source to the X-ray tube to create the same effect.

K-edge filters produce an X-ray beam with a high number of photons in a specific range. The desired energy range is the energy range that is just above the K-absorption edge of the tissue in question. The K-edge is the binding energy of the K-shell electron. This energy level varies from tissue to tissue. The importance of the K-edge is that at photon energies just above this level, the transmission of photons through the tissue in question drops dramatically; that is, the photons are maximally attenuated at this energy level (50). Therefore, to separate bone from soft tissue in a quantifiable fashion, the energy of the photon beam should be just above the K-edge of bone or soft tissue for maximum attenuation. GE Lunar uses a cerium filter in its central devices that has a K-shell absorption edge at 40 keV.* A cerium-filtered X-ray spectrum at 80 kV will contain two photoelectric peaks at about 40 and 70 keV. The samarium K-edge filter employed by Norland in its central devices has a K-shell absorption edge of 46.8 keV. The samarium-filtered X-ray beam at 100 kV produces a low-energy peak at 46.8 keV. In the Norland system, the high-energy peak is variable because the system employs selectable levels of filtration, but the photons are limited to less than 100 keV by the 100 kV employed. The K-edge of both cerium and samarium results in a low-energy peak that approximates the 44-keV low-energy peak of gadolinium-153 used in old dual photon systems.

The Hologic central DXA device utilizes a different system to produce the two photoelectric peaks necessary to separate bone from soft tissue. Instead of employing K-edge filtering of the X-ray beam, Hologic employs alternating pulses to the X-ray source at 70 and 140 kV.

Most regions of the skeleton are accessible with DXA. Studies can be made of the spine in both an anterior-posterior (AP)* and lateral projection. Lumbar spine studies acquired in the lateral projection can elminate the confounding effects of dystrophic calcification on densities measured in the AP direction (51). Lateral scans also eliminate the highly cortical posterior elements, which contribute as much as 47% of the mineral content measured in the AP direction (52). Lateral lumbar spine studies can be limited by rib overlap of L1 and L2 and pelvic overlap of L4, more so when performed in the left lateral decubitus position than the supine position (51,53). Bone density in the proximal femur, forearm, calcaneus, and total body can also be measured with DXA.

---

*A central device is a bone densitometer that can be used to quantify bone density in the spine and proximal femur. The distinction between central and peripheral devices is discussed in detail in Chapter 1.

*Although spine bone density studies with DXA are often referred to as AP spine studies, the beam actually passes in a posterior to anterior direction. Such studies are correctly characterized as PA spine studies, but it has become an accepted convention to refer to them as AP spine bone density studies. The GE Lunar Expert, a fan-array DXA scanner, does acquire spine bone density studies in the AP projection.

Scan times are dramatically shorter with DXA compared to DPA. Early DXA units required approximately 4 minutes for studies of the AP spine or proximal femur. Total body studies required 20 minutes in the medium scan mode and only 10 minutes in the fast scan mode. Newer DXA units scan even faster, with studies of the AP spine or proximal femur requiring less than 1 minute to perform.

The values obtained with dual-energy X-ray studies of the skeleton are highly correlated with values from earlier studies performed with DPA. Consequently, the accuracy of DXA is considered comparable with that of DPA (54–57). DXA spine values and Hologic and Norland DXA proximal femur values are consistently lower than values obtained previously with DPA. There are also differences in the values obtained with DXA equipment from the three major manufacturers.* Values obtained with either a Hologic or Norland DXA unit are consistently lower than those obtained with a Lunar DXA unit, although all are highly correlated with each other (58–60). Comparison studies using all three manufacturers of central DXA devices have resulted in the development of formulas that make it possible to convert values for the lumbar spine and femoral neck obtained on one manufacturer's device to the expected value on another manufacturer's device (see Appendix VII) (61). The margin of error in such conversions is still too great to allow use of such values in following a patient over time, however. Such values should be viewed only as "ball park" figures. Another set of formulas makes possible the conversion of any manufacturer's BMD value at the lumbar spine or total hip to a second value called the "standardized bone mineral density" or sBMD (see Appendix VII) (61,62). The sBMD is always reported in milligrams/square centimeter (mg/cm^2) to distinguish it from the manufacturer's BMD, which is reported in grams/square centimeter (g/cm^2).

Perhaps the most significant advance seen with DXA compared to DPA is the marked improvement in precision. Expressed as a coefficient of variation, short-term precision in normal subjects has been reported as low as 0.9% for the PA lumbar spine and 1.4% for the femoral neck (54). Precision studies over the course of 1 year have reported values of 1% for the PA lumbar spine and 1.7% to 2.3% for the femoral neck (54).

Radiation exposure is extremely low for all types of DXA scans. Expressed as skin dose, radiation exposure during a PA lumbar spine or

---

*See Chapter 1 for a detailed discussion of the difference in values obtained using central devices from different manufacturers, conversion equations, and the development of the standardized BMD (sBMD).

proximal femur study is only 2 to 5 mrem.* The biologically important effective dose or whole-body equivalent dose is only 0.1 mrem *(63)*.

DXA has been used in prospective studies to predict fracture risk. In one of the largest studies of its kind, DXA studies of the proximal femur were demonstrated to have the greatest short-term predictive ability for hip fracture compared to measurements at other sites with SPA or DPA *(17)*.

DXA central devices are called *pencil-beam* or *fan-array* scanners. Examples of pencil-beam scanners are the GE Lunar DPX® Plus, DPX®-L, DPX-IQ™, DPX®-SF, DPX®-A, DPX-MD™, DPX-MD+™ and DPX-NT™; the Hologic QDR® 1000 and QDR® 2000; and the Norland XR-36™, XR-46™, Excell™, and Excell™plus.† Examples of fan-array DXA scanners are the GE Lunar Expert® and Prodigy™; and the Hologic QDR® 4500 A, QDR® 4500 C, QDR® 4500 W, QDR® 4500 SL, and the Delphi™. Figs. 2-9 and 2-10 illustrate the difference between the pencil-beam and fan-array scanners. Pencil-beam scanners employ a collimated or narrowed X-ray beam (narrow like a pencil) that moves in tandem in a rectilinear pattern with the detector or detectors. Fan-array scanners utilize a much broader or fan-shaped beam and an array of detectors, so that an entire scan line can be instantly quantified. Scan times are reduced to as little as 30 seconds for a PA study of the lumbar spine. Image resolution is also enhanced with the fan-array scanners, as shown in the extraordinary images in Fig. 2-11. This has created a new application for bone densitometry scanning called morphometric X-ray absorptiometry (MXA). With MXA, images of the spine obtained in the lateral projection can be used for computer analysis of the vertebral dimensions and diagnosis of vertebral fracture. Fan-array scanners have also been developed to image the lateral spine in its entirety to allow a visual assessment of vertebral size and shape. Examples of scanners with this capability are the Hologic Delphi and the GE Lunar Prodigy. Figures 2-12 and 2-13 are lateral spine images from the GE Lunar Prodigy. In the LVA™ (Lateral Vertebral Assessment) image in Fig. 2-12, a fracture is suggested at T12. In Fig. 2-13, the dimensions of the suspect vertebra are measured with morphometry. Figures 2-14 and 2-15 are IVA™ (Instant Vertebral Assessment) images from the Hologic Delphi. No fractures are apparent in Fig. 2-14. Note the multiple thoracic deformities in Fig. 2-15.

---

*See Chapter 7 for a detailed discussion of radiation dose during DXA studies. See Chapter 4 for a listing of radiation dose according to device and scan type.

†Specific descriptions and photographs of these scanners can be found in Chapter 4.

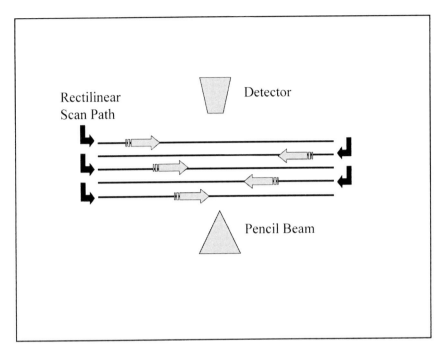

Fig. 2-9. Pencil-beam DXA densitometers. The single detector or sequential detectors move in tandem with the narrowed X-ray beam in a rectilinear scan path.

DXA has effectively replaced DPA in both research and clinical practice. The shortened scan times, improved image resolution, lower radiation dose, improved precision, application to more skeletal sites, and lower cost of operation with DXA have regulated DPA to an honored place in densitometry history.

Peripheral DXA

Dual energy X-ray technology is also being employed in portable devices dedicated to the measurement of one or two appendicular sites. As such, these devices are characterized as peripheral DXA (pDXA) devices. Because these devices employ dual energy X ray, they do not require a water bath or tissue-equivalent gel surrounding the region of the skeleton being studied. As a consequence, they are somewhat easier to maintain and use than SXA devices. Examples of pDXA units are the Lunar PIXI®, the Norland pDEXA®, and the Norland Apollo™, the Schick accuDEXA™, and the Osteometer DexaCare DTX-200. These devices are discussed in detail in Chapter 4.

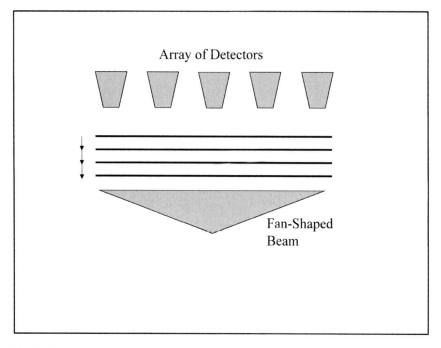

Fig. 2-10. Fan-array DXA densitometers. An array of detectors and fan-shaped beam make possible the simultaneous acquisition of data across an entire scan line.

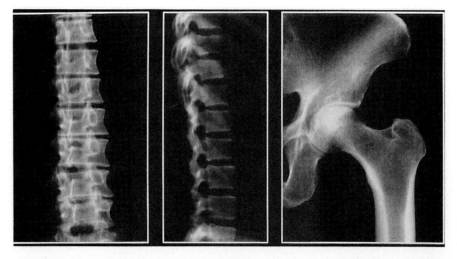

Fig. 2-11. Images from the fan-array imaging densitometer, the GE Lunar EXPERT-XL. (Images courtesy of GE Lunar, Madison, WI.)

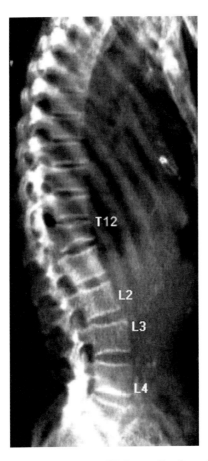

Fig. 2-12. LVA™ image acquired on the GE Lunar Prodigy. A fracture is apparent at T12. (Case courtesy of GE Lunar, Madison, WI.)

Single-Energy X-ray Absorptiometry

Single-energy X-ray absorptiometry (SXA) is the X-ray-based counterpart of SPA, much as DXA is the X-ray-based counterpart of DPA. SXA units were used to measure bone density in the distal radius and ulna and calcaneus. Like their DXA counterparts, SXA units did not utilize radioactive isotopes but did require a water bath or tissue-equivalent gel surrounding the region of the skeleton being measured. The accuracy and precision of SXA were comparable to SPA *(64)*. With the development of portable DXA devices for the measurement of forearm and heel bone density that do not require a water bath or tissue-equivalent gel, SXA is rapidly becoming obsolete, just like its predecessor SPA. The Norland

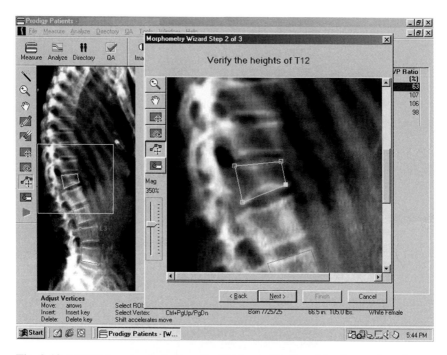

Fig. 2-13. LVA™ image acquired on the GE Lunar Prodigy. Morphometric software allows the user to define the vertebral edges and measure the vertebral heights to quantitatively diagnose fracture. (Case courtesy of GE Lunar, Madison, WI.)

OsteoAnalyzer™ is an SXA device dedicated to heel measurements that is still in use in the United States. It is being phased out, however, in favor of the Norland Apollo™, a dedicated heel DXA device.

Quantitative Computed Tomography

Although quantitative computed tomography (QCT) is a photon absorptiometric technique like SPA, SXA, DPA, and DXA, it is unique in that it provides a three-dimensional or volumetric measurement of bone density and a spatial separation of trabecular from cortical bone. In 1976, Ruegsegger et al. *(65)* developed a dedicated peripheral quantitative CT (pQCT) scanner using ^{125}I for measurements of the radius. Cann and Genant *(66,67)* are credited with adapting commercially available CT scanners for the quantitative assessment of spinal bone density *(66,67)*. It is this approach that has received the most widespread use in the United States, although dedicated CT units for the measurement of the peripheral skeleton, or pQCT units, are in use in clinical centers.

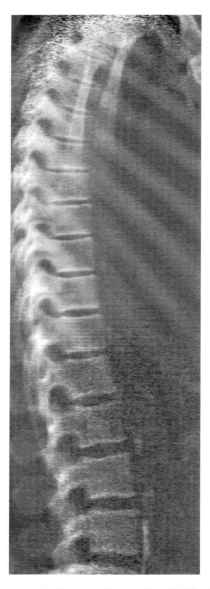

Fig. 2-14. IVA™ image acquired on the Hologic Delphi. No fractures are apparent in the thoracic and lumbar spine although aortic calcification is seen anterior to the lumbar spine. (Case courtesy of Hologic, Bedford, MA.)

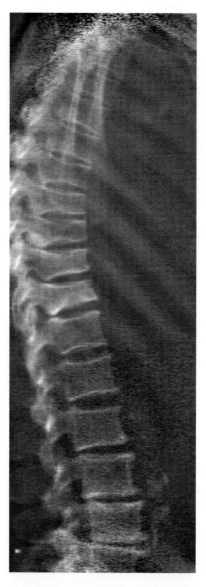

Fig. 2-15. IVA™ image acquired on the Hologic Delphi. There are multiple deformities in the thoracic spine as well as osteophytes in the lower lumbar spine. Aortic calcification is also seen anterior to the lumbar spine. (Case courtesy of Hologic, Bedford, MA.)

QCT studies of the spine utilize a reference standard or phantom that is scanned simultaneously with the patient. The phantom contains varying concentrations of K_2HPO_4 and is placed underneath the patient during the study. A scout view is required for localization and then an 8- to 10-mm-thick slice is measured through the center of two or more vertebral bodies that are generally selected from T12 to L3 *(68)*. A region of interest within the anterior portion of the vertebral body is analyzed for bone density and is reported as milligrams/cubic centimeter K_2HPO_4 equivalents. This region of interest is carefully placed to avoid the cortical shell of the vertebral body. The result is a three-dimensional trabecular density unlike the two-dimensional areal mixed cortical and trabecular densities reported with AP studies of the spine utilizing DPA or DXA.

A study of the spine with QCT requires about 30 minutes *(33)*. The skin radiation dose is generally 100 to 300 mrem. This overestimates the biologically important effective dose because only a small portion of marrow is irradiated during a QCT study of the spine *(63)*. The effective dose or whole-body equivalent dose is generally in the range of only 3 mrem (30 µSv). The localizer scan that precedes the actual QCT study will add an additional 3 mrem to the effective dose. These values are quite acceptable in the context of natural background radiation of approximately 20 mrem per month. Older CT units, which by their design are unable to utilize low kVp settings for QCT studies, may deliver doses 3 to 10 times higher.

The accuracy of QCT for measurements of spine BMD can be affected by the presence of marrow fat *(68–70)*. Marrow fat increases with age, resulting in an increasingly large error in the accuracy of spine QCT measurements in older patients. The accuracy of QCT is reported to range from 5 to 15%, depending on the age of the patient and percentage of marrow fat. The presence of marrow fat results in an underestimation of bone density in the young of about 20 mg/cm^3 and as much as 30 mg/cm^3 in the elderly *(68)*. The error introduced by marrow fat can be partially corrected by applying data on vertebral marrow fat with aging originally developed by Dunnill et al. *(71)*. In an attempt to eliminate the error introduced by marrow fat, dual energy QCT (DEQCT) was developed by Genant and Boyd *(72)*. This method clearly reduced the error introduced by the presence of marrow fat to as low as 1.4% in cadaveric studies *(69,70)*. In vivo, the accuracy with DEQCT is 3 to 6% *(33,68)*. Radiation dose with DEQCT is increased approximately 10-fold compared to regular or single energy QCT (SEQCT), but precision is not as good. The precision of SEQCT for vertebral measurements in expert hands is 1 to 3% and for DEQCT is 3 to 5% *(68,73)*.

The measurement of bone density in the proximal femur with QCT is not readily available. Using both dedicated QCT and standard CT units, investigators have attempted to utilize QCT for measurements of the proximal femur but this capability remains restricted to a few research centers *(74,75)*.

QCT of the spine has been used in studies of prevalent osteoporotic fractures, and it is clear that such measurements can distinguish osteoporotic individuals from normal individuals as well or even better than DPA *(76–79)*. Fractures are rare with values above 110 mg/cc and extremely common below 60 mg/cm^3 *(80)*. Because QCT can isolate and measure trabecular bone, which is more metabolically active than cortical bone, rates of change in disease states observed with QCT spine measurements tend to be greater than those observed with PA spine studies performed with DPA or DXA *(66,81)*. This greater magnitude of change partially offsets the effects of the poorer precision seen with QCT compared to DXA.* The correlations between spine bone density measurements with QCT and skeletal sites measured with other techniques are statistically significant but too weak to allow accurate prediction of bone density at another site from measurement of the spine with QCT *(24,78,79)*. This is no different, however, from attempting to use BMD at the spine obtained with DXA to predict the BMD at other skeletal sites.

Peripheral QCT

Peripheral QCT (pQCT) is becoming more widely available. pQCT devices are utilized primarily for the measurement of bone density in the forearm. Like QCT scans of the spine, pQCT makes possible true three-dimensional or volumetric measurements of bone density in the forearm, which may be particularly useful when the size of the bone is changing, as in pediatric populations. Information on a commercially available pQCT device, the Norland XCT 2000™, can be found in Chapter 4.

QUANTITATIVE ULTRASOUND BONE DENSITOMETRY

Research in quantitative ultrasound (QUS) bone densitometry has been ongoing for more than 40 years. Only in the last few years, however, has

---

*See Chapter 6 for a detailed discussion on the interaction between precision and rate of change in determining the time interval required between measurements to demonstrate significant change.

QUS begun to play a role in the clinical evaluation of the patient. Ultrasound technologies in clinical medicine have traditionally been imaging technologies used, for example, to image the gallbladder or the ovaries. Like photon absorptiometric technologies, however, the application of ultrasound in bone densitometry is not primarily directed at producing an image of the bone. Instead, a quantitative assessment of bone density is desired with the image being secondary in importance.

In theory, the speed with which sound passes through bone is related not only to the density of the bone, but to the quality of the bone as well. Both bone density and bone quality determine a bone's resistance to fracture. Therefore, the speed of sound through bone can be related to the risk of fracture. These relationships can be illustrated mathematically. For example, the bone's ability to resist fracture *(R)* can be described as the amount the bone deforms when it is subjected to a force *(F)* that is moderated by the bone's ability to resist that force, the elastic modulus *(E)*, as shown in Eq. 1:

$$R = F/E \tag{1}$$

Studies have shown that the elastic modulus, E, is determined by both bone density and bone quality. Mathematically this is represented in Eq. 2, in which K is a constant representing bone quality and ρ represents bone density:

$$E = K\rho^2 \tag{2}$$

From such an equation, it becomes clear that the bone's ability to resist a force and not fracture is determined by changes in bone density and bone quality. When ultrasound passes through a material, the velocity of the sound wave is also related to the elastic modulus and density of the material, as shown in Eq. 3.

$$V = \sqrt{E/\rho} \tag{3}$$

When Eqs. 2 and 3 are combined, it becomes clear that the velocity of ultrasound through bone is directly related to the square root of the product of bone density and bone quality.

$$V = \sqrt{K\rho^2/\rho} \tag{4}$$
$$V = \sqrt{K\rho} \tag{5}$$

The velocity with which ultrasound passes through normal bone is quite fast and varies depending upon whether the bone is cortical or trabecular. Speeds of 3000 to 3600 m/sec are typical in cortical bone, with speeds of 1650–2300 m/sec typical of trabecular bone.

To calculate velocity, ultrasound densitometers must measure the distance between two points and the time required for the sound wave to travel between these two points. Similar to the reporting of BMD when it is the BMC and area that are actually measured, a major reported ultrasound parameter is speed of sound (SOS), although it is time and distance that are actually measured. Higher values of SOS indicate greater values of bone density.

A second ultrasound parameter is broadband ultrasound attenuation (BUA). This parameter is reported in decibels per megahertz (dB/MHz). BUA is perhaps best understood using the analogy of a child's toy such as a slinky. When the toy is stretched out and then suddenly released, the energy imparted to the rings by stretching them causes the rings to oscillate for a period of time, with the oscillations becoming progressively less and then finally stopping as the energy is lost. The same thing happens to the sound wave as it passes through bone. Some of the energy is lost from the sound wave and the oscillations of the sound wave are diminished. How much energy is lost is again related to the density of the bone and to the architecture. Like SOS, higher BUA values indicate greater bone density.

Most devices report both SOS and BUA. However, one manufacturer has mathematically combined SOS and BUA into a proprietary index called the Stiffness Index. Another manufacturer reports an estimated BMD that is derived from the measurements of SOS and BUA. QUS devices are considered peripheral devices and are generally quite portable. They employ no ionizing radiation, unlike their SXA or DXA peripheral counterparts. The calcaneus is the most common skeletal site assessed with QUS, but devices exist that can be applied to the radius, finger, and tibia. In heel QUS measurements, heel width apparently has little if any effect on BUA but may have a slight effect on SOS (82). Most ultrasound devices require some type of coupling medium between the transducers and the bone. This is often accomplished by placing the heel into a water bath, but ultrasound gel is also used for heel measurements and measurements at other skeletal sites. Systems that utilize water baths are called *wet systems* and systems that utilize gel are called *dry systems.* The GE Lunar Achilles+™, GE Lunar Achilles Express™, Sunlight Omnisense™ 7000S, Quidel QUS-2™, Norland McCue C.U.B.A. Clinical™, Hologic Sahara™ Clinical Bone Sonometer, and Osteometer Ultrasure DTU-one are all examples of QUS densitometers currently available for clinical use. These devices are discussed in more detail in Chapter 4.

The technical differences among devices from various manufacturers are even greater than those seen with DXA devices. Different frequency ranges and transducer sizes may be employed from device to device. Within the same skeletal site, slightly different regions of interest may be measured. Consequently, values obtained on one QUS device are not necessarily comparable with values obtained on another QUS device.

The physics of ultrasound suggest that it should provide information about the bone that goes beyond a simple measurement of mass or density. Clinical research has tended to confirm this assumption, although perhaps not to the extent that was originally hoped. In a very large study of 5662 older women, both SOS and BUA predicted the risk of hip fracture as well or better than did measurements of BMD at the femoral neck using DXA *(83)*. Similar findings were reported in the Study of Osteoporotic Fractures by Bauer et al. *(84)*.

REFERENCES

1. Dennis, J. (1897) A new system of measurement in X-ray work. *Dental Cosmos* **39**, 445–454.
2. Price, W. A. (1901) The science of dental radiology. *Dental Cosmos* **43**, 483–503.
3. Johnston, C. C. and Epstein, S. (1981) Clinical, biochemical, radiographic, epidemiologic, and economic features of osteoporosis. *Orthop. Clin. North Am.* **12**, 559–569.
4. (1984) Measurement of bone mass and turnover, in *Osteoporosis in Clinical Practice* (Aitken, M., ed.), John Wright & Sons, Bristol, pp. 19, 20.
5. Singh, J., Nagrath, A. R., Maini, P. S. (1970) Changes in trabecular pattern of the upper end of the femur as an index of osteoporosis. *J. Bone Joint Surg. Am.* **52-A**, 457–467.
6. Bohr, H. and Schadt, O. (1983) Bone mineral content of femoral bone and lumbar spine measured in women with fracture of the femoral neck by dual photon absorptiometry. *Clin. Orthop.* **179**, 240–245.
7. Nordin, B. E. C. (1983) Osteoporosis with particular reference to the menopause, in *The Osteoporotic Syndrome* (Avioli, L. V., ed.), Grune & Stratton, New York, pp. 13–44.
8. Shimmins, J., Anderson, J. B., Smith D. A., et al. (1972) The accuracy and reproducibility of bone mineral measurements "in vivo." (a) The measurement of metacarpal mineralisation using an X-ray generator. *Clin. Radiol.* **23**, 42–46.
9. Exton-Smith, A. N., Millard, P. H., Payne, P. R., Wheeler, E. F. (1969) Method for measuring quantity of bone. *Lancet* **2**, 1153, 1154.
10. Dequeker, J. (1982) Precision of the radiogrammetric evaluation of bone mass at the metacarpal bones, in *Non-invasive Bone Measurements: Methodological Problems* (Dequeker, J. and Johnston, C. C., eds.), IRL, Oxford, pp. 27–32.
11. Aitken, J. M., Smith, C. B., Horton, P. W., et al. (1974) The interrelationships between bone mineral at different skeletal sites in male and female cadavera. *J. Bone Joint Surg. Br.* **56B**, 370–375.
12. Meema, H. E. and Meindok, H. (1992) Advantages of peripheral radiogrammetry over dual-photon absorptiometry of the spine in the assessment of prevalence of osteoporotic vertebral fractures in women. *J. Bone Miner. Res.* **7**, 897–903.

13. Bywaters, E. G. L. (1948) The measurement of bone opacity. *Clin. Sci.* **6**, 281–287.
14. Barnett, E. and Nordin, B. E. C. (1961) Radiologic assessment of bone density. 1.-The clinical and radiological problem of thin bones. *Br. J. Radiol.* **34**, 683–692.
15. Mack, P. B., Brown, W. N., Trapp, H. D. (1949) The quantitative evaluation of bone density. *Am. J. Roentgenol. Rad. Ther.* **61**, 808–825.
16. Vose, G. P. and Mack, P. B. (1963) Roentgenologic assessment of femoral neck density as related to fracturing. *Am. J. Roentgenol. Rad. Ther. Nucl. Med.* **89**, 1296–1301.
17. Cummings, S. R., Black, D. M., Nevitt, M. C., et al. (1993) Bone density at various sites for prediction of hip fractures. *Lancet* **341**, 72–75.
18. Mazess, R. B. (1983) Noninvasive methods for quantitating trabecular bone, in *The Osteoporotic Syndrome* (Avioli, L.V., ed.), Grune & Stratton, New York, pp. 85–114.
19. Mack, P. B., O'Brien, A. T., Smith, J. M., Bauman, A. W. (1939) A method for estimating degree of mineralization of bones from tracings of roentgenograms. *Science* **89**, 467.
20. Mack, P. B. and Vogt, F. B. (1971) Roentgenographic bone density changes in astronauts during representative Apollo space flight. *Am. J. Roentgenol. Rad. Ther. Nucl. Med.* **113**, 621–633.
21. Cosman, F., Herrington, B., Himmelstein, S., Lindsay, R. (1991) Radiographic absorptiometry: a simple method for determination of bone mass. *Osteoporos. Int.* **2**, 34–38.
22. Yates, A. J., Ross, P. D., Lydick, E., Epstein, R. S. (1995) Radiographic absorptiometry in the diagnosis of osteoporosis. *Am. J. Med.* **98**, 41S–47S.
23. Yang, S., Hagiwara, S., Engelke, K., et al. (1994) Radiographic absorptiometry for bone mineral measurement of the phalanges: precision and accuracy study. *Radiology* **192**, 857–859.
24. Kleerekoper, M., Nelson, D. A., Flynn, M. J., Pawluszka, A. S., Jacobsen, G., Peterson, E. L. (1994) Comparison of radiographic absorptiometry with dual-energy X-ray absorptiometry and quantitative computed tomography in normal older white and black women. *J. Bone Miner. Res.* **9**, 1745–1749.
25. Mussolino, M. E., Looker, A. C., Madans, J. H., Edelstein, D., Walker, R. E., Lydick, E., Epstein, R. S., Yates, A. J. (1997) Phalangeal bone density and hip fracture risk. *Arch. Intern. Med.* **157**, 433–438.
26. Huang, C., Ross, P. D., Yates, A. J., Walker, R. E., Imose, K., Emi, K., Wasnich, R.D. (1998) Prediction of fracture risk by radiographic absorptiometry and quantitative ultrasound: a prospective study. *Calcif. Tissue Int.* **6**, 380–384.
27. Cameron, J. R. and Sorenson, G. (1963) Measurements of bone mineral in vivo: an improved method. *Science* **142**, 230–232.
28. Vogel, J. M. (1987) Application principles and technical considerations in SPA, in *Osteoporosis Update 1987* (Genant, H. K, ed.), University of California Printing Services, San Francisco, pp. 219–231.
29. Johnston, C. C. (1983) Noninvasive methods for quantitating appendicular bone mass, in *The Osteoporotic Syndrome* (Avioli, L. V., ed.), Grune & Stratton, New York, pp. 73–84.
30. Barden, H. S. and Mazess, R. B. (1989) Bone densitometry of the appendicular and axial skeleton. *Top. Geriatric Rehabil.* **4**, 1–12.
31. Kimmel, P. L. (1984) Radiologic methods to evaluate bone mineral content. *Ann. Intern. Med.* **100**, 908–911.
32. Steiger, P. and Genant, H. K. (1987) The current implementation of single-photon absorptiometry in commercially available instruments, in *Osteoporosis Update 1987*

(Genant, H. K., ed.), University of California Printing Services, San Francisco, pp. 233–240.

33. Chesnut, C. H. (1993) Noninvasive methods for bone mass measurement, in *The Osteoporotic Syndrome*, 3rd ed. (Avioli, L., ed.), Wiley-Liss, New York, pp. 77–87.

34. Gardsell, P., Johnell, O., Nilsson, B. E. (1991) The predictive value of bone loss for fragility fractures in women: a longitudinal study over 15 years. *Calcif. Tissue Int.* **49**, 90–94.

35. Hui, S. L., Slemenda, C. W., Johnston, C. C. (1989) Baseline measurement of bone mass predicts fracture in white women. *Ann. Intern. Med.* **111**, 355–361.

36. Ross, P. D., Davis, J. W., Vogel, J. M., Wasnich, R. D. (1990) A critical review of bone mass and the risk of fractures in osteoporosis. *Calcif. Tissue Int.* **46**, 149–161.

37. Melton, L. J., Atkinson, E. J., O'Fallon, W. M., Wahner, H. W., Riggs, B. L. (1993) Long-term fracture prediction by bone mineral assessed at different skeletal sites. *J. Bone Miner. Res.* **8**, 1227–1233.

38. Black, D. M., Cummings, S. R., Genant, H. K., Nevitt, M. C., Palermo, L., Browner, W. (1992) Axial and appendicular bone density predict fracture in older women. *J. Bone Miner. Res.* **7**, 633–638.

39. Nord, R. H. (1987) Technical considerations in DPA, in *Osteoporosis Update 1987* (Genant, H.K., ed.), University of California Printing Services, San Francisco, pp. 203–212.

40. Dunn, W. L., Wahner, H. W., Riggs, B. L. (1980) Measurement of bone mineral content in human vertebrae and hip by dual photon absorptiometry. *Radiology* **136**, 485–487.

41. Reed, G. W. (1966) The assessment of bone mineralization from the relative transmission of [241]Am and ^{137}Cs radiations. *Phys. Med. Biol.* **11**, 174.

42. Roos, B. and Skoldborn, H. (1974) Dual photon absorptiometry in lumbar vertebrae. I. Theory and method. *Acta Radiol. Ther. Phys. Biol.* **13**, 266–290.

43. Mazess, R. B., Ort, M., Judy, P. (1970) Absorptiometric bone mineral determination using [153]Gd, in *Proceedings of Bone Measurements Conference* (Cameron, J. R., ed.), U.S. Atomic Energy Commission, pp. 308–312.

44. Wilson, C. R. and Madsen, M. (1977) Dichromatic absorptiometry of vertebral bone mineral content. *Invest. Radiol.* **12**, 180–184.

45. Madsen, M., Peppler, W., Mazess, R. B. (1976) Vertebral and total body bone mineral content by dual photon absorptiometry. *Calcif. Tissue Res.* **2**, 361–364.

46. Wahner, W. H., Dunn, W. L., Mazess, R. B., et al. (1985) Dual-photon Gd-153 absorptiometry of bone. *Radiology* **156**, 203–206.

47. Lindsay, R., Fey, C., Haboubi, A. (1987) Dual photon absorptiometric measurements of bone mineral density increase with source life. *Calcif. Tissue Int.* **41**, 293, 294.

48. Cummings, S. R. and Black, D. B. (1986) Should perimenopausal women be screened for osteoporosis? *Ann. Intern. Med.* **104**, 817–823.

49. Drinka, P. J., DeSmet, A. A., Bauwens, S. F., Rogot, A. (1992) The effect of overlying calcification on lumbar bone densitometry. *Calcif. Tissue Int.* **50**, 507–510.

50. Curry, T. S., Dowdey, J. E., Murry, R. C. (1990) *Christensen's Physics of Diagnostic Radiology,* Lea & Febiger, Philadelphia.

51. Rupich, R. C., Griffin, M. G., Pacifici, R., Avioli, L. V., Susman, N. (1992) Lateral dual-energy radiography: artifact error from rib and pelvic bone. *J. Bone Miner. Res.* **7**, 97–101.

52. Louis, O., Van Den Winkel, P., Covens, P., Schoutens, A., Osteaux, M. (1992) Dual-energy X-ray absorptiometry of lumbar vertebrae: relative contribution of body and

posterior elements and accuracy in relation with neutron activation analysis. *Bone* **13,** 317–320.

53. Peel, N. F. A., Johnson, A., Barrington, N. A., Smith, T. W. D., Eastell, R. (1993) Impact of anomalous vertebral segmentation of measurements of bone mineral density. *J. Bone Miner. Res.* **8,** 719–723.

54. Lees, B. and Stevenson, J. C. (1992) An evaluation of dual-energy X-ray absorptiometry and comparison with dual-photon absorptiometry. *Osteoporos. Int.* **2,** 146–152.

55. Kelly, T. L., Slovik, D. M., Schoenfeld, D. A., Neer, R. M. (1988) Quantitative digital radiography versus dual photon absorptiometry of the lumbar spine. *J. Clin. Endocrinol. Metab.* **76,** 839–844.

56. Holbrook, T. L., Barrett-Connor, E., Klauber, M., Sartoris, D. (1991) A population-based comparison of quantitative dual-energy X-ray absorptiometry with dual-photon absorptiometry of the spine and hip. *Calcif. Tissue Int.* **49,** 305–307.

57. Pouilles, J. M., Tremollieres, F., Todorovsky, N., Ribot, C. (1991) Precision and sensitivity of dual-energy X-ray absorptiometry in spinal osteoporosis. *J. Bone Miner. Res.* **6,** 997–1002.

58. Laskey, M. A., Cirsp, A. J., Cole, T. J., Compston, J. E. (1992) Comparison of the effect of different reference data on Lunar DPX and Hologic QDR-1000 dual-energy X-ray absorptiometers. *Br. J. Radiol.* **65,** 1124–1129.

59. Pocock, N. A., Sambrook, P. N., Nguyen, T., Kelly, P., Freund, J., Eisman, J. (1992) Assessment of spinal and femoral bone density by dual X-ray absorptiometry: comparison of Lunar and Hologic instruments. *J. Bone Miner. Res.* **7,** 1081–1084.

60. Lai, K. C., Goodsitt, M. M., Murano, R., Chesnut, C. C. (1992) A comparison of two dual-energy X-ray absorptiometry systems for spinal bone mineral measurement. *Calcif. Tissue Int.* **50,** 203–208.

61. Genant, H. K., Grampp, S., Gluer, C. C., Faulkner, K. G., Jergas, M., Engelke, K., Hagiwara, S., Van Kuijk, C. (1994) Universal standardization for dual X-ray absorptiometry: patient and phantom cross-calibration results. *J. Bone Miner. Res.* **9,** 1503–1514.

62. Hanson, J. (1997) Standardization of femur BMD. *J. Bone Miner. Res.* **12,** 1316, 1317.

63. Kalender, W. A. (1992) Effective dose values in bone mineral measurements by photon-absorptiometry and computed tomography. *Osteoporos. Int.* **2,** 82–87.

64. Kelly, T. L., Crane, G., Baran, D. T. (1994) Single x-ray absorptiometry of the forearm: precision, correlation, and reference data. *Calcif. Tissue Int.* **54,** 212–218.

65. Ruegsegger, P., Elsasser, U., Anliker, M., Gnehn, H., Kind, H., Prader, A. (1976) Quantification of bone mineralisation using computed tomography. *Radiology* **121,** 93–97.

66. Genant, H. K., Cann, C. E., Ettinger, B., Gorday, G. S. (1982) Quantitative computed tomography of vertebral spongiosa: a sensitive method for detecting early bone loss after oophorectomy. *Ann. Intern. Med.* **97,** 699–705.

67. Cann, C. E. and Genant, H. K. (1980) Precise measurement of vertebral mineral content using computed tomography. *J. Comput. Assist. Tomogr.* **4,** 493–500.

68. Genant, H. K., Block, J. E., Steiger, P, Gluer, C. (1987) Quantitative computed tomography in the assessment of osteoporosis, In *Osteoporosis Update 1987,* (Genant, H. K., ed.), University of California Printing Services, San Francisco, pp. 49–72.

69. Laval-Jeantet, A. M., Roger, B., Bouysse, S., Bergot, C., Mazess, R. B. (1986) Influence of vertebral fat content on quantitative CT density. *Radiology* **159,** 463–466.

70. Reinbold, W, Adler, C. P., Kalender, W. A., Lente, R. (1991) Accuracy of vertebral mineral determination by dual-energy quantitative computed tomography. *Skel. Radiol.* **20,** 25–29.

71. Dunnill, M. S., Anderson, J. A., Whitehead, R. (1967) Quantitative histological studies on age changes in bone. *J. Pathol. Bacteriol.* **94**, 274–291.
72. Genant, H. K. and Boyd, D. (1977) Quantitative bone mineral analysis using dual energy computed tomography. *Invest. Radiol.* **12**, 545–551.
73. Cann, C. E. (1987) Quantitative computed tomography for bone mineral analysis: technical considerations, in *Osteoporosis Update 1987* (Genant, H. K., ed.), University of California Printing Services, San Francisco, pp. 131–144.
74. Sartoris, D. J., Andre, M., Resnick, C., Resnick, D. (1986) Trabecular bone density in the proximal femur: quantitative CT assessment. *Radiol.* **160**, 707–712.
75. Reiser, U. J. and Genant, H. K. (1984) Determination of bone mineral content in the femoral neck by quantitative computed tomography, 70th Scientific Assembly and Annual Meeting of the Radiological Society of North America, Washington, DC.
76. Gallagher, C., Golgar, D., Mahoney, P., McGill, J. (1985) Measurement of spine density in normal and osteoporotic subjects using computed tomography: relationship of spine density to fracture threshold and fracture index. *J. Comput. Assist. Tomogr.* **9**, 634, 635.
77. Raymaker, J. A., Hoekstra, O., Van Putten, J., Kerkhoff, H., Duursma, S.A. (1986) Osteoporosis fracture prevalence and bone mineral mass measured with CT and DPA. *Skel. Radiol.* **15**, 191–197.
78. Reinbold, W. D., Reiser, U. J., Harris, S. T., Ettinger, B., Genant, H. K. (1986) Measurement of bone mineral content in early postmenopausal and postmenopausal osteoporotic women: a comparison of methods. *Radiology* **160**, 469–478.
79. Sambrook, P. N., Bartlett, C., Evans, R., Hesp, R., Katz, D., Reeve, J. (1985) Measurement of lumbar spine bone mineral: a comparison of dual photon absorptiometry and computed tomography. *Br. J. Radiol.* **58**, 621–624.
80. Genant, H. K., Ettinger, B., Harris, S. T., Block, J. E., Steiger, P. (1988) Quantitative computed tomography in assessment of osteoporosis, in *Osteoporosis: Etiology, Diagnosis and Management,* (Riggs, B. L. and Melton, L. J., eds.) Raven, New York, pp. 221–249.
81. Richardson, M. L., Genant, H. K., Cann, C. E., et al. (1985) Assessment of metabolic bone disease by quantitative computed tomography. *Clin. Orthop. Rel. Res.* **195**, 224–238.
82. Njeh, C. F., Boivin, C. M., Langton, C. M. (1997) The role of ultrasound in the assessment of osteoporosis: a review. *Osteoporos. Int.* **7**, 7–22.
83. Hans, D., Dargent-Molina, P., Schott, A. M., et al. (1996) Ultrasonographic heel measurements to predict hip fracture in elderly women: the EPIDOS prospective study. *Lancet* **348**, 511–514.
84. Bauer, D. C., Gluer, C. C., Cauley, J. A., et al. (1997) Bone ultrasound predicts fractures strongly and independently of densitometry in older women: a prospective study. *Arch. Intern. Med.* **157**, 629–634.

3 Skeletal Anatomy in Densitometry

CONTENTS

THE SPINE IN DENSITOMETRY

Studies of the lumbar spine performed with dual photon absorptiometry (DPA) or dual energy X-ray absortiometry (DXA) are generally acquired by the passage of photon energy from the posterior to anterior direction. They are properly characterized as being posteroanterior (PA) spine studies. These studies, nevertheless, are often referred to as anterior-posterior (AP) spine studies, probably as a holdover from plain films of the lumbar spine that are acquired in the AP projection. The GE Lunar Expert®, a fan-array scanner, does acquire lumbar spine bone density images in the

61

AP direction. Compared to plain radiography, however, the beam direction in a DXA study of the spine has less influence on the appearance of the image and no influence on the measured bone mineral content (BMC) or bone minerals density (BMD). Studies of the lumbar spine may also be acquired in the lateral projection using DXA. Such studies may be performed with the patient supine or in the left lateral decubitus position, depending on the type of DXA unit being employed.

Vertebral Anatomy

The whole vertebra can be divided into two major components: the body and the posterior elements. The posterior elements consist of the pedicles, the lamina, the spinous process, the transverse processes, and the inferior and superior articulating surfaces. The appearance of the image of the spine on an AP or PA study is predominantly determined by the relative density of the various elements that make up the entire vertebra. Figure 3-1A is a photograph of a posterior view of the lumbar spine with the intervertebral discs removed. Figures 3-1B,C demonstrates the appearance of the spine as the transverse processes are removed and then when the vertebral bodies are removed. What remains in Fig. 3-1C is characteristic of the appearance of the lumbar spine on a PA DXA lumbar spine study. The transverse processes are eliminated from the scan field, and the vertebral bodies are not well seen because they are both behind and equally or less dense than the posterior elements. In a study of 34 lumbar vertebrae taken from 10 individuals, age 61 to 88, the mineral content of the posterior elements averaged 47% of the mineral content of the entire vertebrae (1).

The posterior elements that remain in Fig. 3-1C form the basis of the DXA lumbar spine image as seen in Fig. 3-2. The unique shapes of the posterior elements of the various lumbar vertebrae have led to the use of these shapes as an aid in the identification of the lumbar vertebrae. L1, L2, and L3 are often characterized as having a U- or Y-shaped appearance. L4 is described as looking like a block H or X. L5 has the appearance of a block I on its side. Figure 3-3 is a graphic illustration of these shapes. Compare these shapes to the actual posterior elements seen in Fig. 3-1C and the DXA lumbar spine study shown in Fig. 3-2. Although the transverse processes are generally not seen on a spine bone density study, the processes at L3 will sometimes be partially visible, since this vertebra tends to have the largest transverse processes. Figures 3-4 A and B are the spine images only from the study shown in Fig. 3-2. In Fig. 3-4B, the shapes of the posterior elements have been outlined for emphasis.

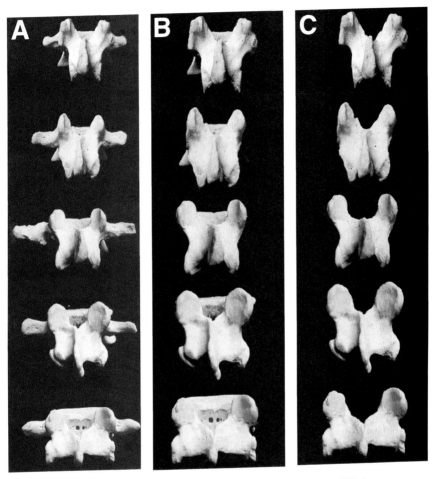

Fig. 3-1. Lumbar spine in the posterior view. **(A)** Intact vertebrae; **(B)** the transverse processes have been removed; **(C)** the vertebral bodies have been removed, leaving only the posterior elements. (Adapted from McMinn, R. M. H., Hutchings, R. T., Pegington, J., and Abrahams, P. H. [1993] *Colour Atlas of Human Anatomy*, 3rd ed., p. 83. By permission of Mosby.)

On PA or AP DXA lumbar spine studies, L1 through L4 are quantified. Although L5 can be seen, it is not usually quantified because of interference from the pelvis. L1 frequently has the lowest BMC and BMD of the four lumbar vertebrae measured *(2)*. In a study of 148 normal women age 50–60, Peel et al. *(2)* found that the BMC increased between L1–L2, L2–L3, and L3–L4 although the increase between L3–L4 was roughly half that seen at the other levels, as shown in Table 3-1. BMD increased

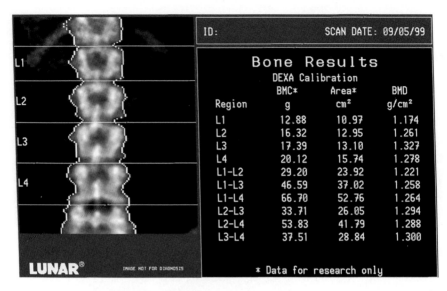

	ID:		SCAN DATE: 09/05/99

Bone Results

DEXA Calibration

Region	BMC* g	Area* cm²	BMD g/cm²
L1	12.88	10.97	1.174
L2	16.32	12.95	1.261
L3	17.39	13.10	1.327
L4	20.12	15.74	1.278
L1-L2	29.20	23.92	1.221
L1-L3	46.59	37.02	1.258
L1-L4	66.70	52.76	1.264
L2-L3	33.71	26.05	1.294
L2-L4	53.83	41.79	1.288
L3-L4	37.51	28.84	1.300

LUNAR® IMAGE NOT FOR DIAGNOSIS * Data for research only

Fig. 3-2. DXA PA spine study acquired on the GE Lunar DPX®. The shapes of the vertebrae in this image are primarily created by the posterior elements. The shapes in this study are classic. The expected increase in BMC and area is also seen from L1 to L4. The increase in BMD from L1 to L3, with a decline from L3 to L4, is also typical.

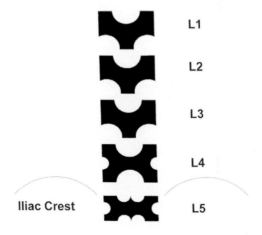

L1

L2

L3

L4

Iliac Crest   L5

Fig. 3-3. Graphic illustration of the characteristic shapes of the lumbar vertebrae as seen on a DXA PA spine study.

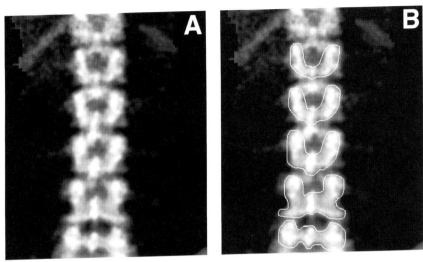

Fig. 3-4. (A) DXA PA spine image acquired on the GE Lunar DPX. This is the spine image from the study shown in Fig. 3-2, with the intervertebral disk markers and bone-edge markers removed for clarity. **(B)** The shapes have been outlined for emphasis.

Table 3-1
Incremental Change in BMC and BMD Between Adjacent
Vertebrae in 148 Normal Women Ages 50–60 as Measured by DXA

Vertebrae	Increase in BMC (g)	Increase in BMC (%)	Increase in BMD (g/cm²)	Increase in BMD (%)
L1–L2	2.07	13.7	0.090	7.9
L2–L3	2.43	14.8	0.050	4.3
L3–L4	1.13	5.0	−0.004[a]	−0.8[a]

[a]Not statistically significant.
Reprinted from *Journal of Bone and Mineral Research* 1993;8:719–723 with permission from the American Society for Bone and Mineral Research.

between L1–L2 and L2–L3 but showed no significant change between L3–L4. The average change between L3–L4 was actually a decline of 0.004 g/cm². The largest increase in BMD occurred between L1–L2. The apparent discrepancies in the magnitude of the change in BMC and BMD between the vertebrae are the result of the progressive increase in area of the vertebrae from L1 to L4. The DXA PA lumbar spine study shown in Fig. 3-2 illustrates the progressive increase in BMC and area from L1

Table 3-2
Percentage of Women with Various Combinations
of Numbers of Lumbar Vertebrae and Position of Lowest Ribs

No. of lumbar vertebrae	Position of lowest ribs	Women (%)
5	T12	83.5
5	T11	7.2
4	T12	2.1
4	T11	5.3
6	T12	1.1
6	L1	0.8

Reprinted from *Journal of Bone and Mineral Research* 1993;8:719–723 with permission from the American Society for Bone and Mineral Research.

to L4 and the expected pattern of change in BMD between the vertebral levels.

Studies from both Peel et al. *(2)* and Bornstein and Peterson *(3)* suggest that the majority of individuals have five lumbar vertebrae with the lowest set of ribs on T12. Bornstein and Peterson *(3)* found that only 17% of 1239 skeletons demonstrated a pattern of vertebral segmentation and rib placement other than five lumbar vertebrae with the lowest ribs on T12. Similarly, Peel et al. found something other than the expected pattern of five lumbar vertebrae with the lowest ribs on T12 in only 16.5% of 375 women. An additional 7.2% had five lumbar vertebrae but had the lowest level of ribs on T11. Therefore, 90.7% of the women studied by Peel et al. *(2)* had five lumbar vertebrae. Only 1.9% (or 7) women had six lumbar vertebrae. In three of these women ribs were seen on L1. This was the only circumstance in which ribs were seen on L1. Of the entire group, 7.5% had only four lumbar vertebrae. In the majority of cases here, the lowest ribs were seen on T11. Table 3-2 summarizes these findings.

Knowledge of the frequency of anomalous vertebral segmentation, the characteristic shapes created by the posterior elements on a PA lumbar spine bone density study, and the expected incremental change in BMC and BMD can be used to label the vertebrae correctly. If the vertebrae are mislabeled, comparisons to the normative databases will be misleading. The expected effect of mislabeling T12 as L1 is a lowering of the BMC or BMD at L1, which would then compare unfavorably to the reference value for L1. The BMC and BMD averages for L1–L4 or L2–L4 would also be lowered. The degree to which BMC is lowered by mislabeling is substantially greater than BMD, as shown in Table 3-3 *(2)*. The assumption

Table 3-3
Effect of Mislabeling T12 as L1 on BMC
and BMD in AP DXA Spine Measurements

Measurement	Difference	Mean %
BMC		
L1	1.61 g	11.5
L2–L4	3.47 g	8.4
L1–L4	4.8 g	8.4
BMD		
L2–L4	0.035 g/cm²	3.6
L1–L4	0.039 g/cm²	3.5

Reprinted from *Journal of Bone and Mineral Research* 1993;8:719–723 with permission from the American Society for Bone and Mineral Research.

that the lowest set of ribs is found at the level of T12 is often used as the basis for labeling the lumbar vertebrae. As can be seen from Table 3-2, this assumption would result in the vertebrae being labeled incorrectly in 13.3% of the population. As a consequence, all the aforementioned criteria should be employed in determining the correct labeling of the lumbar vertebrae. This should obviate the need for plain films for the sole purpose of labeling the vertebrae in the vast majority of instances. Figure 3-5 is a PA spine study in which the labeling of the lumbar vertebra was not straightforward. The characteristic shapes of the vertebrae are easily seen, but ribs are not projecting from what should be T12. The labeling shown in Fig. 3-5 is correct.

PA and AP lumbar spine bone density measurements are extremely useful in predicting fracture risk and following the effects of a variety of disease processes and therapeutic interventions. Unfortunately, the lumbar spine is also the site most commonly affected by structural changes or artifacts that may affect either the accuracy or precision of the measurement or both.

Artifacts in PA or AP Spine Densitometry

VERTEBRAL FRACTURES

Any type of vertebral fracture is expected to cause an increase in the BMD at the site of the fracture. Because DXA measurements of the lumbar spine are often employed in patients with osteoporosis, osteoporotic fractures in the lumbar spine are a common problem, rendering the

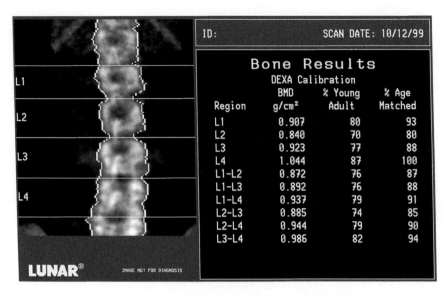

Fig. 3-5. DXA PA spine study acquired on the GE Lunar DPX. The vertebra labeled L4 has a classic block H or X shape. However, no ribs are seen protruding from the vertebra that should be T12. It is far more likely that this represents five lumbar vertebrae with the lowest ribs on T11 than six lumbar vertebrae with the lowest ribs on T12. Also note that the BMD at L1 is higher than at L2, which is unusual. A lateral lumbar spine X ray of this patient, shown in Fig. 3-7, confirmed a fracture at L1.

measurement of BMD inaccurate if the fractured vertebrae are included. An increased precision error would also be expected if the fractured vertebrae were included in BMD measurements performed as part of a serial evaluation of BMD. Although a fractured lumbar vertebra can be excluded from consideration in the analysis of the data, this reduces the maximum number of contiguous vertebrae in the lumbar spine that are available for analysis. For reasons of statistical accuracy and precision, the average BMD for three or four contiguous vertebrae is preferred over averages of two vertebrae or the BMD of a single vertebra. Figure 3-6 illustrates a PA lumbar spine study in which a fracture was apparent at L3. Although the BMD at L3 is expected to be higher than either L2 or L4, it is disproportionately higher. The L2–L4 BMD average will be increased because of the effect of the fracture on the BMD at L3. In the DXA PA lumbar spine study shown in Fig. 3-5, the image does not as readily suggest a fracture. The BMD at L1, however, is higher than the BMD at L2, which is unusual. A plain lateral film of the lumbar spine of this patient, shown in Fig. 3-7, confirmed a fracture at L1.

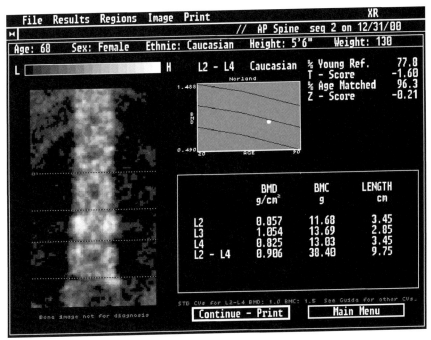

Fig. 3-6. DXA PA spine study acquired on the Norland XR-36®. The image suggests a loss of vertebral height and increased sclerosis at L3. Although the BMD at L3 is expected to be higher than at L2, the BMD at L3 here is markedly higher. These findings suggest a fracture at this level, but this must be confirmed. In any case, the L2–L4 BMD will be increased by this structural change. (Case courtesy of Norland Medical Systems, Ft. Atkinson, WI.)

Other structural changes within the spine can affect BMD measurements. Osteophytes and facet sclerosis can increase BMD when measured in the AP or PA projection. Aortic calcification will also potentially affect the BMD when measured in the AP or PA spine because the X-ray beam will detect the calcium in the aorta as it passes through the body on an anterior-to-posterior or posterior-to-anterior path. It is therefore useful to note how often these types of changes are expected in the general population and the potential magnitude of the effect these changes may have on the measured BMD in the lumbar spine.

EFFECTS OF OSTEOPHYTES ON BMD

In 1982, Krolner et al. *(4)* observed that in subjects with osteophytes, a statistically significant increase in the BMD was observed in the AP

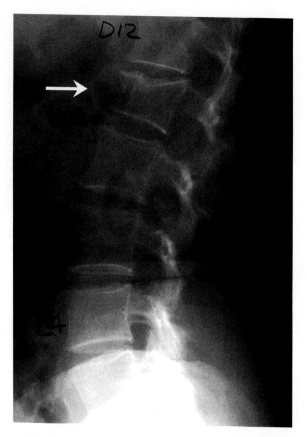

Fig. 3-7. Lateral lumbar spine X ray of the patient whose DXA study is shown in Fig. 3-5. The arrow indicates a fracture at L1.

spine when compared with control subjects without osteophytes. More recently, Rand et al. *(5)* evaluated a population of 144 postmenopausal women ages 40 to 84, with an average age of 63.3, for the presence of osteophytes, scoliosis, and aortic calcification. These were generally healthy women referred for the evaluation of BMD because of suspected postmenopausal osteoporosis. Table 3-4 lists the percentages of these women found to have these types of degenerative changes. Based on these findings, Rand et al. *(5)* estimated the likelihood of degenerative changes in the spine as being less than 10% in women under the age of 50. In 55-year-old women, however, the likelihood jumped to 40%, and in 70 year-old-women, to 85%. Of these types of degenerative changes, however, only the presence of osteophytes significantly increased the BMD.

Table 3-4
Frequency of Specific Types of Degenerative Changes
in Spines of 144 Women Ages 40–84

Type of degenerative change	% with Change (n)
Osteophytes	45.8 (66)
Osteochondrosis	21.5 (31)
Vascular calcification	24.3 (35)
Scoliosis	22.2 (32)
Any type	59.0 (72)

Adapted with permission of the publisher from Rand, T., Seidl, G., Kainberger, F., et al. Impact of spinal degenerative changes on the evaluation of bone mineral density with dual energy X-ray absorptiometry (DXA). *Calcif. Tissue Int.* 1997;60:430–433.

The magnitude of the increase caused by the osteophytes ranged from 9.5% at L4 to 13.9% at L1. Cann et al. *(6)* also estimated the increase in BMD from osteophytes in the spine at 11%. In 1997, Liu et al. *(7)* studied 120 men and 314 women, ages 60 to 99. Lumbar spine osteophytes were found in 75% of the men and 61.1% of the women. The effect of osteophytes on the BMD was sufficiently great to cause 50% of the men and 25% of the women with osteopenia to be misdiagnosed. About 20% of the men and 10% of the women with osteoporosis were misdiagnosed because of the effect of osteophytes on the BMD.

In Fig. 3-8, osteophytes are clearly visible at L2 on the lateral lumbar radiograph. The appearance of this region on the DXA PA lumbar spine study in Fig. 3-9 suggests a sclerotic process at this level. Osteophytes and end-plate sclerosis are also seen on the plain film in Fig. 3-10. The effect on the DXA image of the lumbar spine, shown in Fig. 3-11, is dramatic. There is also an obvious increase in the BMD at L2 and L3.

EFFECTS OF AORTIC CALCIFICATION ON BMD

Although it did not significantly increase BMD, vascular calcification was seen in 24.3% of the population studied by Rand et al. *(5)* In a study of aortic calcification in 200 women age 50 or older by Frye et al. *(8)*, the percentage of women with aortic calcification and the effect on BMD measured in the PA lumbar spine was noted. A grading system for both linear calcifications and calcified plaques was applied to lateral spine films with a grade of 0 indicating neither type of calcification and a grade of 2 indicating the most severe degree. Figure 3-12 shows the percentage of women with any degree of aortic calcification and severe (grade 2)

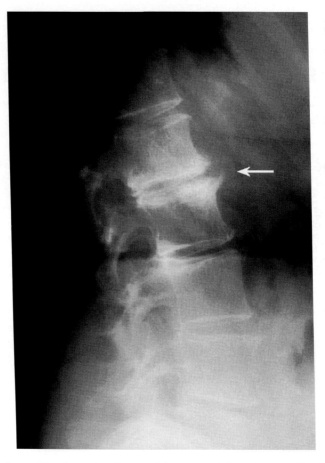

Fig. 3-8. Lateral lumbar spine X ray of the patient whose DXA study is shown in Fig. 3-9. The arrow indicates a region of end-plate sclerosis and osteophyte formation.

calcification. The percentage with any degree of aortic calcification was extremely low under age 60 but did increase dramatically in women age 60 and older. The percentage of women with severe aortic calcification, however, remained low throughout the 50s, 60s, and 70s. Even in women age 80 and older, the percentage did not exceed 30%. Table 3-5 summarizes the effect on BMD in women with any degree of aortic calcification and severe aortic calcification. Neither effect was statistically significant. These findings are similar to those of Frohn et al. *(9)*, Orwoll et al. *(10)*, Reid et al. *(11)*, Banks et al. *(12)*, and Drinka et al. *(13)*, in which no significant effect of aortic calcification was seen on the BMD measured

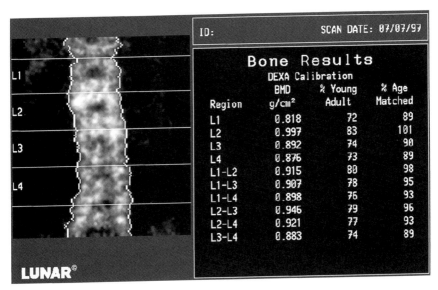

	ID:		SCAN DATE: 07/07/97	

Bone Results

DEXA Calibration

Region	BMD g/cm²	% Young Adult	% Age Matched
L1	0.818	72	89
L2	0.997	83	101
L3	0.892	74	90
L4	0.876	73	89
L1-L2	0.915	80	98
L1-L3	0.907	78	95
L1-L4	0.898	76	93
L2-L3	0.946	79	96
L2-L4	0.921	77	93
L3-L4	0.883	74	89

LUNAR©

Fig. 3-9. DXA PA spine study acquired on the GE Lunar DPX. The image suggests a sclerotic process at L2. The BMD is also increased more than expected in comparison to L1 and is higher than L3, which is unusual. These findings are compatible with the end-plate sclerosis and osteophytes seen in Fig. 3-8.

in the PA spine. The studies from Orwoll et al. *(10)* and Drinka et al. *(13)* were performed in men.

Aortic calcification is not easily seen on most DXA PA lumbar spine studies. In Fig. 3-13A, however, the faint outline of the calcified aorta is visible. The aorta is easily seen on the lateral DXA image in Fig. 3-13B. Figure 3-14 shows both studies. In this case, the DXA lateral spine study can be used to eliminate the effects of the calcified aorta on the BMD measurement.

EFFECTS OF FACET SCLEROSIS ON BMD

Unlike aortic calcification, facet sclerosis can have a profound effect on the measured BMD in the AP or PA projection. In the study by Drinka et al. *(13)* noted earlier, 113 elderly men were evaluated with standard AP and lateral lumbar spine films and DPA of the lumbar spine. A grading system for facet sclerosis was developed with a grade of 0 indicating no sclerosis and a grade of 3 indicating marked sclerosis. As shown in Table 3-6, grade 1 sclerosis had no significant effect on the BMD. Grades 2

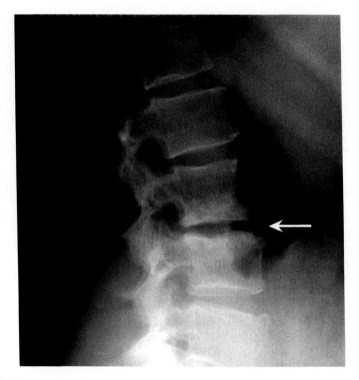

Fig. 3-10. Lateral lumbar spine X ray of the patient whose DXA study is shown in Fig. 3-11. The arrow indicates a region of marked end-plate sclerosis.

and 3, however, markedly increased the BMD at the vertebral levels at which the facet sclerosis was found. Figure 3-15 is a PA spine BMD study in which facet sclerosis is suggested at L3 by the appearance of the image. The BMD values at L3 and L4 are also markedly higher than expected based on the values at L1 and L2. The plain film of this patient shown in Fig. 3-16 confirms facet sclerosis at the lower lumbar levels.

OTHER CAUSES OF ARTIFACTS IN PA AND AP LUMBAR SPINE STUDIES

There are other potential causes of apparent increases in the BMD in the AP or PA lumbar spine. Stutzman et al. *(14)* identified pancreatic calcifications, renal stones, gallstones, contrast agents, and ingested calcium tablets in addition to osteophytes, aortic calcification, and fractures as possible causes of error. Figures 3-17, 3-18, and 3-19 illustrate other

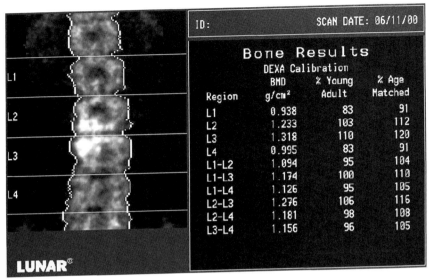

Fig. 3-11. DXA PA spine study acquired on the GE Lunar DPX. The image dramatically suggests the sclerotic process seen on the X ray in Fig. 3-10. There is a marked increase in the BMD at L2 and L3 compared with L1 and L4.

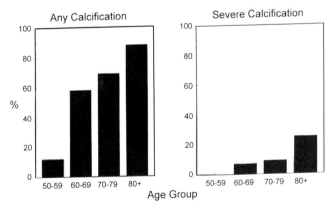

Fig. 3-12. Prevalence of aortic calcification in women age 50 and over. (Reprinted from Frye, M. A., Melton, L. J., Bryant, S. C. et al. Osteoporosis and calcification of the aorta. *Bone Miner.* 1992;19:185–194, with kind permission from Elsevier Science Ireland, Bay 15K, Shannon Industrial Estate, Co., Clare, Ireland.)

Table 3-5
Effect of Aortic Calcification on BMD in Spine

| Site | BMD | | | |
	Observed	Expected	Difference	Expected %
BMD spine				
Any grade 1 or 2	0.93	0.92	0.01	101.4
Any grade 2	0.94	0.89	0.05	106.7

Adapted from Frye, M. A., Melton, L. J., Bryant, S. C. et al. Osteoporosis and calcification of the aorta. *Bone Min.* 1992;19:185–194, with kind permission from Elsevier Science Ireland, Bay 15K, Shannon Industrial Estate, Co., Clare, Ireland.

structural changes in the spine that will affect the BMD measured in the PA projection.

The Spine in the Lateral Projection

The effect on BMD measured in the AP or PA projection from aortic calcification, facet sclerosis, osteophytes, and other degenerative changes in the spine can be overcome by quantifying the bone density of the spine in the lateral projection, as shown in Fig. 3-14. In addition, the highly cortical posterior elements and a portion of the cortical shell of the vertebral body can be eliminated from the measurement, resulting in a more trabecular measure of bone density in the spine. This is desirable in those circumstances in which a trabecular measure of bone density is indicated, and particularly in circumstances in which changes in trabecular bone are being followed over time. The higher metabolic rate of trabecular bone compared with that of cortical bone should result in a much larger magnitude of change in this more trabecular measure of bone density compared to the mixed cortical-trabecular measure of bone density in the PA spine. The measurement of bone density by DXA in the lateral projection is not a measurement of 100% trabecular bone because all the cortical vertebral shell cannot be eliminated from analysis.

Vertebral identification in the lateral projection can be difficult. The lumbar vertebrae are generally identified by the relative position of the overlapping pelvis and the position of the lowest set of ribs. The position of the pelvis tends to differ, however, when the study is performed in the left lateral decubitus position compared with the supine position. Rupich et al. *(15)* found that the pelvis overlapped L4 in only 15% of individuals when studied in the supine position. Jergas et al. *(16)* reported a figure

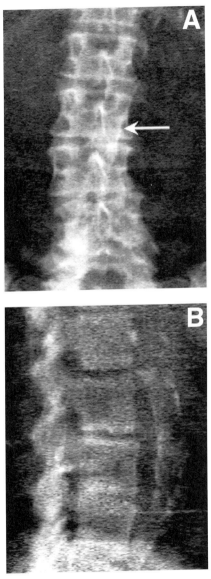

Fig. 3-13. PA and lateral DXA lumbar spine images acquired on the Hologic QDR®
4500. The arrow seen in (**A**) indicates the faint outline of the calcified aorta that is
easily seen on the lateral study in (**B**). (Case courtesy of Hologic, Bedford, MA.)

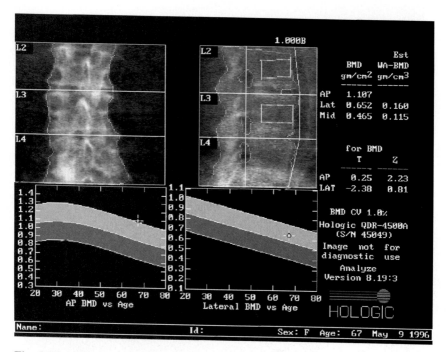

Fig. 3-14. DXA PA and lateral lumbar spine study acquired on the Hologic QDR 4500. These are the analyzed studies for the images shown in Fig. 3-13. (Case courtesy of Hologic, Bedford, MA.)

of 19.7% for L4 overlap for individuals studied in the supine position. In DXA studies performed in the left lateral decubitus position, Peel et al. *(2)* found that pelvic overlap of L4 occurred in 88% of individuals. In the other 12%, the pelvis overlapped L5 in 5% and the L3–L4 disc space or L3 itself in 7%. Consequently, while the position of the pelvis tends to identify L4 in most individuals scanned in the left lateral decubitus position, it also eliminates the ability to accurately measure the BMD at L4 in those individuals. The ribs are less useful than the pelvis in identifying the lumbar vertebrae. Rib overlap of L1 can be expected in the majority of individuals, whether they are studied in the supine or left lateral decubitus position (2). This may not be seen, however, in the 12.5% of individuals whose lowest set of ribs is on T11.

While the location of the pelvis and the presence of rib overlap aid in identification of the vertebrae, they also limit the available vertebrae for analysis. When a lateral spine DXA study is performed in the left lateral decubitus position, L4 cannot be analyzed in the majority of individuals because of pelvic overlap. L1 is generally not analyzed because of rib

Table 3-6
Increase in BMD from Facet Sclerosis

	Grade 2	Grade 3
L1	0.275	0.465
L2	0.312	0.472
L3	0.184	0.343
L4	0.034	0.247
Average	0.201	0.382

Values are in grams/square centimeter.
Adapted with permission of the publisher from Drinka PJ, DeSmet, A. A., Bauwens, S. F., et al. The effect of overlying calcification on lumbar bone densitometry. *Calcifi. Tissue Int.* 1992;50:507–510.

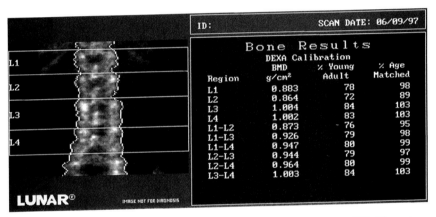

Fig. 3-15. DXA PA lumbar spine study acquired on the GE Lunar DPX. There is a marked increase in the BMD between L2 and L3, which is maintained at L4. The image faintly suggests sclerosis in the region of the facet joints at L3 and L4. This is more dramatically seen in the plain film of this patient shown in Fig. 3-16.

overlap, regardless of whether the study is performed supine or in the left lateral decubitus position. Rupich et al. *(15)* also found rib overlap of L2 in 90% of individuals studied in the supine position. It was estimated that rib BMC added 10.4% to the L2 BMC. Thus, when lateral DXA studies are performed in the left lateral decubitus position, L3 may be the only vertebra that is not affected by either pelvic or rib overlap. In the supine position, L3 and L4 are generally unaffected. This means that depending on the positioning required by the technique, the value from a single vertebra or from only a two-vertebrae average may have to be

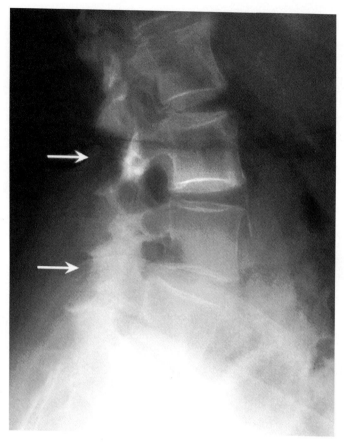

Fig. 3-16. Lateral lumbar spine X ray of the patient whose bone density study is shown in Fig. 3-15. The arrows indicate sclerotic regions in the posterior elements.

used. This is undesirable, although sometimes unavoidable, from the standpoint of statistical accuracy and precision.

If the vertebrae are misidentified in the lateral projection, the effect on BMD can be significant. In the study by Peel et al. *(2)*, misidentification of the vertebral levels would have resulted in 12% of individuals in whom the pelvis did not overlap L4 in the left lateral decubitus position. If L2 was misidentified as L3, the BMD of L3 was underestimated by an average of 5.7%. When L4 was misidentified as L3, the BMD at L3 was overestimated by an average of 3.1%. Although spine X rays are rarely justified for the sole purpose of vertebral identification on a DXA study performed in the PA or AP projection, this may occasionally be required for DXA lumbar spine studies performed in the lateral projection. Analysis

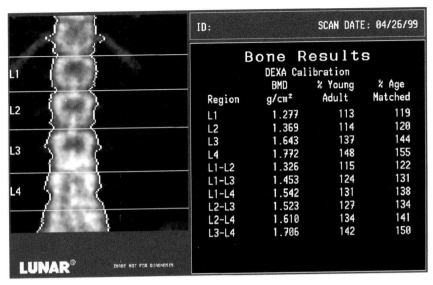

ID:			SCAN DATE: 04/26/99

Bone Results

DEXA Calibration

Region	BMD g/cm²	% Young Adult	% Age Matched
L1	1.277	113	119
L2	1.369	114	120
L3	1.643	137	144
L4	1.772	148	155
L1-L2	1.326	115	122
L1-L3	1.453	124	131
L1-L4	1.542	131	138
L2-L3	1.523	127	134
L2-L4	1.610	134	141
L3-L4	1.706	142	150

LUNAR® IMAGE NOT FOR DIAGNOSIS

Fig. 3-17. DXA PA lumbar spine study acquired on the GE Lunar DPX. The image suggests increased density at L3 and L4, but there is also a linear vertical lucency over L4. The BMD values are markedly increased at L3 and L4. This patient had previously undergone an L3–L4, L4–L5 interbody fusion and laminectomy at L4. Although the laminectomy alone would decrease the BMD at L4, the fusion mass has increased the BMD at L3 and L4 dramatically.

may be restricted to only one or two vertebrae because of rib and pelvic overlap. This reduces the statistical accuracy and precision of the measurement. Because of this reduction in accuracy, consideration should be given to combining lateral DXA spine studies with bone density assessments of other sites for diagnostic purposes.

THE PROXIMAL FEMUR IN DENSITOMETRY

Proximal Femur Anatomy

Figure 3-20 shows the gross anatomy of the proximal femur. In densitometry, the proximal femur has been divided into specific regions of interest (ROIs). The proximal femur study shown in Fig. 3-21 illustrates these regions, which are based on the anatomy shown in Fig. 3-20. Ward's area is a region with which most physicians and technologists are not familiar. Ward's triangle, as it was originally called, is an anatomic region in the neck of the femur that is formed by the intersection of three

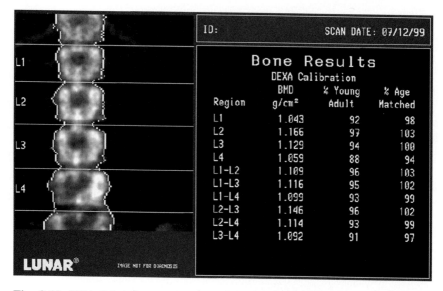

Fig. 3-18. DXA PA spine study acquired on the GE Lunar DPX. The image is unusual at L4, with what appears to be an absence of part of the posterior elements. This was confirmed with plain films and should decrease the BMD at L4.

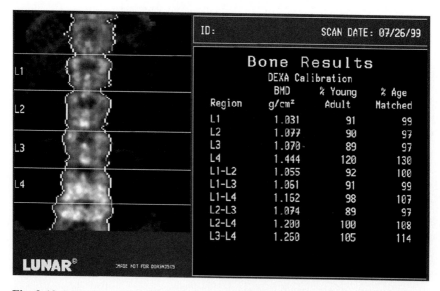

Fig. 3-19. DXA PA spine study acquired on the GE Lunar DPX. The image suggests a marked sclerotic reaction at L4 and L5. There is also a marked increase in the BMD at L4, compared with L3. This sclerotic process was thought to be the result of an episode of childhood disciitis. The patient was asymptomatic.

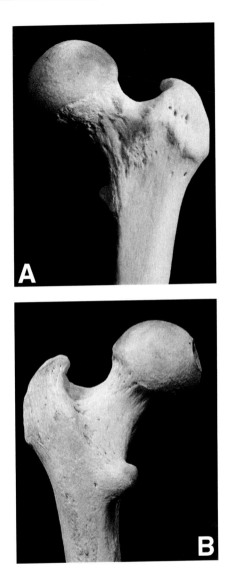

Fig. 3-20. (A) Proximal femur as viewed from the front. The lesser trochanter is behind the shaft of the femur. **(B)** Proximal femur as viewed from behind. The lesser trochanter is clearly seen to be a posterior structure. (Adapted from McMinn, R. M. H., Hutchings, R. T., Pegington, J., et al. [1993] *Colour Atlas of Human Anatomy,* 3rd ed., pp. 267, 268. By permission of Mosby.)

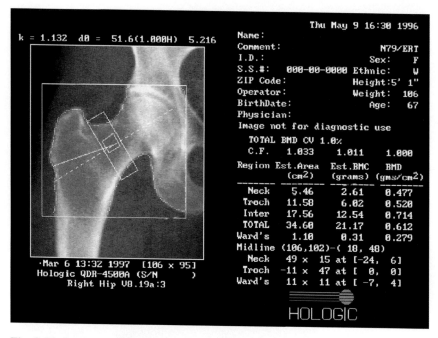

Fig. 3-21. A DXA proximal femur study acquired on the Hologic QDR® 4500. Five ROIs are defined in this study. (Case courtesy of Hologic, Bedford, MA.)

trabecular bundles, as shown in Fig. 3-22. In densitometry, Ward's triangle is a calculated region of low density in the femoral neck rather than a specific anatomic region. Because the region in densitometry is identified as a square, the region is generally now called Ward's area, instead of Ward's triangle. The total femur ROI encompasses all the individual regions: femoral neck, Ward's area, trochanteric region, and shaft. Each of these regions within this one bone contains a different percentage of trabecular and cortical bone, as noted in Table 1-2 in Chapter 1.

Effects of Rotation on BMD in the Proximal Femur

The lesser trochanter is an important anatomic structure from the perspective of recognizing the degree to which the femur has been rotated during positioning for a proximal femur bone density study. Precision in proximal femur bone density testing is highly dependent on reproduction of the degree of rotation of the proximal femur from study to study. In positioning the patient for a proximal femur study, internally rotating the femur 15 to 20° will bring the femoral neck parallel to the plane of the

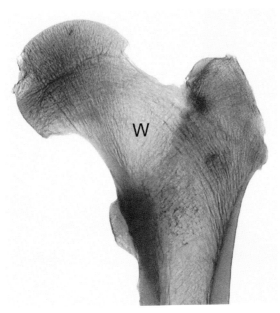

Fig. 3-22. Ward's triangle, indicated by the letter *W*, is formed by the intersection of bundles of trabeculae in the femoral neck. (Adapted from McMinn, R. M. H., Hutchings, R. T., Pegington, J., Abraham, P. H., et al. [1993] *Colour Atlas of Human Anatomy*, 3rd ed., p. 271. By permission of Mosby.)

scan table. This rotation is accomplished with the aid of positioning devices provided by the manufacturers. In this position, BMD values in the femoral neck are the lowest. If the femoral neck rotation is increased or decreased from this position, the femoral neck BMD value will increase. Table 3-7 illustrates the magnitude of the increase in BMD in a cadaver study from Goh et al. *(17)*. The apparent length of the neck of the femur will decrease as rotation is increased or decreased from the basic position. When the neck of the femur is parallel to the plane of the scan table, the X-ray beam passes through the neck at a 90° angle to the neck. With changes in rotation, the neck is no longer parallel to the scan table and the beam enters the neck at an angle that is greater or lesser than 90°. The result is an apparent shortening of the length of the neck and an increase in the mineral content in the path of the beam. The combination results in an apparent increase in BMD. The only visual clue to consistent rotation is the reproduction of the size and shape of the lesser trochanter. Because the trochanter is a posterior structure, leg positioning in which the femur has not been rotated sufficiently internally tends to produce a

Table 3-7
Effect of Increasing Internal or External Rotation
from Neutral Position on Femoral Neck BMD (gm/cm^2) of Cadaveric Femurs

	Neutral	External rotation from neutral of			Internal rotation from neutral of		
Cadaver no.	0°	15°	30°	45°	15°	30°	45°
1	0.490	0.524	0.549	0.628	0.510	0.714	0.845
2	0.574	0.567	0.632	0.711	0.581	0.619	0.753
3	0.835	0.872	0.902	1.071	0.874	1.037	1.222
4	0.946	0.977	1.005	1.036	1.102	1.283	1.492

Reproduced with permission of the publisher from Goh, J. C. H., Low, S. L., Bose, K. Effect of femoral rotation on bone mineral density measurements with dual energy X-ray absorptiometry. *Calcif. Tissue Int.* 1995;57:340–343.

very large and pointed lesser trochanter. Excessive internal rotation of the proximal femur will result in total disappearance of the lesser trochanter.

The size of the lesser trochanter in the DXA proximal femur image in Fig. 3-23A indicates correct internal rotation. This can be compared with the size of the lesser trochanter seen in the DXA proximal femur study in Fig. 3-23B. The lesser trochanter is very large and pointed, indicating insufficient internal rotation. Although this would be undesirable in a baseline study of the proximal femur, follow-up studies using the proximal femur in this patient should be done with this same degree of rotation. Any change in rotation from the baseline study would be expected to affect the magnitude of change in the BMD, decreasing the precision of the study.

Effects of Leg Dominance on BMD in the Proximal Femur

In general, there does not seem to be a significant difference in the BMD in the regions of the proximal femur between the right and left legs of normal individuals *(18,19)*. Leg dominance, unlike arm dominance, does not appear to exert a significant effect on the bone densities in the proximal femur and is not used to determine which femur should be studied.

Effects of Scoliosis, Osteoarthritis, Osteophytes, Surgery, and Fracture on BMD in the Proximal Femur

Structural changes and artifacts that interfere with DXA proximal femoral BMD measurements occur less often than at the spine. Osteoarthritic

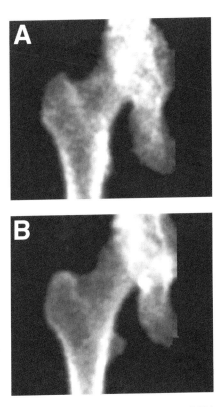

Fig. 3-23. Images of the proximal femur acquired during DXA studies on the Lunar DPX. **(A)** The lesser trochanter is clearly seen but is small and rounded, indicating proper internal rotation of the proximal femur during positioning. Compare this lesser trochanter to the lesser trochanter seen in **(B).** This is the same patient seen in (A), but here the proximal femur was not rotated internally, sufficiently causing the lesser trochanter to appear large and pointed.

change in the hip joint may cause thickening of the medial cortex and hypertrophy of the trabeculae in the femoral neck, which may increase the BMD in the femoral neck and Ward's area *(20)*. The trochanteric region apparently is not affected by such change and has been recommended as the preferred site to evaluate in patient's with osteoarthritis of the hip *(21)*. Osteophytes in the proximal femur are apparently much less common than osteophytes in the lumbar spine *(7)*. They also appear to have little effect on the bone densities measured in the proximal femur. In patients with scoliosis, however, lower bone densities have been reported on the side of the convexity *(22)*. If a worst-case measurement is desired, the bone density in the proximal femur should be measured in the femur on the side of the convexity. Fracture of the proximal femur and surgically implanted prostheses will render measurements of bone density in the proximal femur inaccurate.

If osteoarthritis or some other process restricts the ability of the patient to rotate the femur properly, the study should not be done. An attempt should be made to scan the opposite proximal femur if possible. Similarly, if pain restricts the patient's range of motion such that the femur cannot be properly positioned, the study should not be done because the results will be not be valid.

THE FOREARM IN DENSITOMETRY

Nomenclature

The nomenclature used to describe the various sites in the forearm that are assessed with densitometry is confusing. Commonly measured sites are the 33% or ⅓ site, the 50%, and 10% sites, the 5-mm and 8-mm sites, and the ultradistal site.* The sites designated by a percentage are named based on the location of the site in relationship to the overall length of the ulna. This is true for the site regardless of whether the site is on the ulna or the radius. In other words, the 50% site on the radius is located at a site on the radius that is directly across from the site on the ulna that marks 50% of the overall ulnar length, not 50% of the overall radial length. The 5-mm and 8-mm sites are located on either bone at the point where the separation distance between the radius and ulna is 5 or 8 mm, respectively. In Fig. 3-24, the approximate location of these sites is indicated. The 33% and 50% sites are both characterized as proximal radial sites, and the 10% site is considered a distal site. The ultradistal site is variously centered at a distance of either 4 or 5% of the ulnar length. There is nothing inherent in the definition of distal, ultradistal, and proximal, however, that specifies the exact location of sites bearing these names. In Figs. 3-25, 3-26, 3-27, and 3-28, the location of variously named ROIs from several different DXA forearm devices can be compared.

The clinically important difference among these sites is the relative percentages of cortical and trabecular bone found at the site. Table 1-3 in Chapter 1 summarizes the percentages of cortical and trabecular bone at the various sites on the radius. These values are transferable to sites at the same location on the ulna.

---

*Although a mathematical conversion of ⅓ to a percentage would result in a value of 33.3%, the site when named as a percentage is called the 33% site

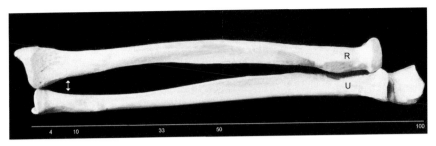

Fig. 3-24. Forearm. The scale at the bottom of the figure indicates ulnar length. The numbers reflect the percentage of ulnar length at which commonly measured sites are centered on either bone. The arrow between the two bones indicates the 8-mm separation point. R, radius; U, ulna. (Adapted from McMinn, R. M. H., Hutchings, R. T., Pegington, J., et al. [1993] *Colour Atlas of Human Anatomy*, 3rd ed., p. 110. By permission of Mosby.)

Effects of Arm Dominance on Forearm BMD

Unlike the proximal femur, arm dominance has a pronounced effect on the bone density in the forearm. In healthy individuals, the BMC at the 33% radial site differs by 6% to 9% between the dominant and nondominant arms *(23)*. A difference of 3% has been reported at the 8-mm site *(24)*. If the individual is involved in any type of repetitive activity that involves unilateral arm activity, the difference between the dominant and nondominant arm densities will be magnified to an even greater extent. Two studies of tennis players, an activity in which the dominant arm is subjected to repeated loading and impact, illustrated the effect of unilateral activity. In a study by Huddleston et al. *(25)* the BMC in the dominant forearm at the 50% radial site measured by single photon absorptiometry (SPA) was 13% greater than in the nondominant arm. In a more recent study from Kannus et al. *(26)* using DXA, the side-to-side difference in BMD in tennis players averaged 10.8% at the distal radius and 9.9% at the mid radius. The corresponding values in the non-tennis-playing control subjects were only 3.4 and 2.5%, respectively. Because of these recognized differences, the nondominant arm has traditionally been studied when the bone content or density is being quantified for the purposes of diagnosis or assessment of fracture risk. Most reference databases for the machines in current use have been created using the nondominant arm. Comparisons of the dominant arm to these reference databases would not be valid.

---

and is located on the radius or forearm at a location that represents 33%, not 33.3%, of the length of the ulna.

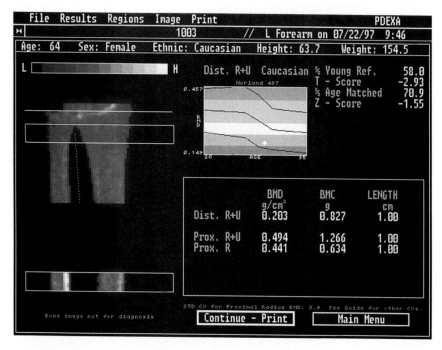

Fig. 3-25. DXA study of the forearm acquired on the Norland pDEXA®. Note the location of the ROIs called distal (dist.) and proximal (prox.). BMD values are given for the radius and ulna combined at both regions and for the radius alone at the proximal ROI.

Some manufacturers supply databases for the dominant arm that can be used for comparisons if the dominant arm is to be studied. The operator's manual for the densitometry device should be consulted to determine which arm was used to create the database(s) provided by the manufacturer.

Effects of Artifacts on BMD in the Forearm

The forearm sites are relatively free from the confounding effects of most of the types of artifacts that are often seen in the lumbar spine. The presence of a prior fracture in the forearm will affect the BMC or BMD measurements in the forearm close to the prior fracture site. A study from Akesson et al. *(27)* suggested that in women with a prior fracture of the distal radius, the BMC was increased by 20% at the distal radius of the fractured arm in comparison with the nonfractured arm, irrespective of arm dominance. It is obviously important for the technologist to ask whether the patient has experienced a prior wrist or forearm fracture.

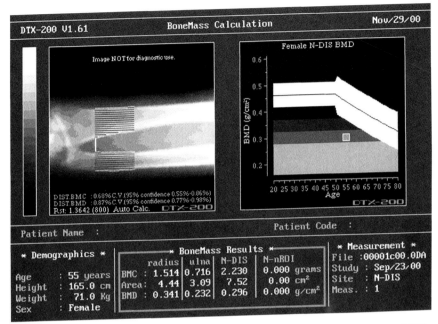

Fig. 3-26. DXA study of the forearm acquired on the Osteometer DexaCare DTX-200. The ROI is called the distal (DIS) region and begins at the 8-mm separation point. Values are given for each bone and for both bones combined. This distal ROI is not the same as the distal region of interest shown in Fig. 3-25.

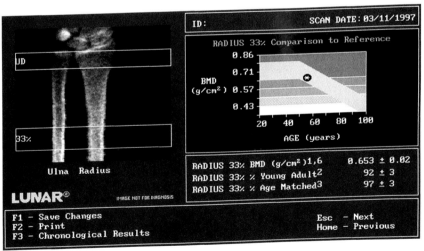

Fig. 3-27. DXA study of the forearm acquired on the GE Lunar DPX. The two primary ROIs are the ultradistal (UD) and 33% regions. These are similar but not identical in location to the distal and proximal regions seen in the study in Fig. 3-25.

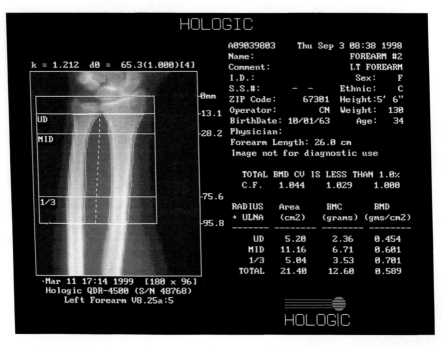

Fig. 3-28. DXA study of the forearm acquired on the Hologic QDR 4500. Three ROIs are shown. An ultradistal (UD), mid-, and ⅓ ROI are indicated. The ⅓ ROI is located similarly to the 33% ROI shown in Fig. 3-27. Note that the midregion here is clearly not located at a point that would correspond to 50% of ulnar length. It is between the ultradistal and ⅓ sites.

Unfortunately, Akesson et al. *(27)* also noted that in a group of older women who were known to have previously had a distal radial fracture, many of the women did not recall the fracture or incorrectly recalled which arm was fractured. It was noted, however, that the forearm most often fractured was the dominant forearm.

THE METACARPALS, PHALANGES, AND CALCANEUS

Other skeletal sites can be studied using the techniques available today. The metacarpals, phalanges, and calcaneus were among the very first sites studied with the older techniques of radiographic photodensitometry and radiogrammetry. These sites are increasingly utilized today with the advent of computerized radiographic absorptiometry, computerized radiogrammetry, and peripheral DXA and ultrasound units that measure these sites.

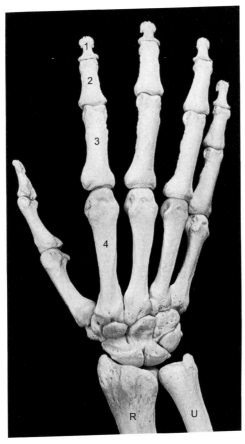

Fig. 3-29. Dorsal surface of the hand. The numbering on the index finger would apply to the long, ring, and small fingers as well. 1, 2, and 3: distal, mid-, and proximal phalanges, respectively; 4: metacarpal; R and U: radius and ulna, respectively. (Adapted from McMinn, R. M. H., Hutchings, R. T., Pegington, J, et al. [1993] *Colour Atlas of Human Anatomy*, 3rd ed., p. 112. By permission of Mosby.)

Figure 3-29 illustrates the anatomy of the hand and the location of the metacarpals and phalanges. The middle phalanges of the index, long, and ring fingers are the phalangeal regions most often quantified today. Figure 3-30 illustrates the appearance of the phalanges on a computerized radiographic absorptiometry study, and Fig. 3-31 illustrates the appearance of the metacarpals on a computer-assisted radiogrammetry study. The calcaneus is commonly called the heel; the anatomy is illustrated in Fig. 3-32. The calcaneus contains an extremely high percentage of trabecular bone and is exquisitely sensitive to weight-bearing activities. Both the

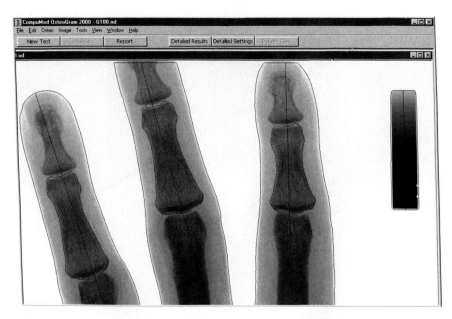

Fig. 3-30. Radiographic absorptiometry analysis of the midphalanges of the index, long, and ringer fingers. (Case provided courtesy of CompuMed, Los Angeles, CA.)

phalanges and the calcaneus have been shown to be useful sites for the prediction of hip fracture risk *(28–30)*. The relative percentages of trabecular and cortical bone are noted for the phalanges and calcaneus in Tables 1-2 and 1-3 in Chapter 1.

REFERENCES

1. Louis, O., Van Den Winkel, P., Covens, P., Schoutens, A., Osteaux, M. (1992) Dual-energy X-ray absorptiometry of lumbar vertebrae: relative contribution of body and posterior elements and accuracy in relation with neutron activation analysis. *Bone* **13,** 317–320.
2. Peel, N. F. A., Johnson, A., Barrington, N. A., Smith, T. W. D., Eastell, R. (1993) Impact of anomalous vertebral segmentation of measurements of bone mineral density. *J. Bone Miner. Res.* **8,** 719–723.
3. Bornstein, P. E. and Peterson, R. R. (1966) Numerical variation of the presacral vertebral column in three population groups in North America. *Am. J. Phys. Anthropol.* **25,** 139–146.
4. Krolner, B., Berthelsen, B., Nielsen, S. P. (1982) Assessment of vertebral osteopenia— comparison of spinal radiography and dual-photon absorptiometry. *Acta Radiol. Diagn.* **23,** 517–521.
5. Rand, T., Seidl, G., Kainberger, F., Resch, A., Hittmair, K., Schneider, B., Gluer,

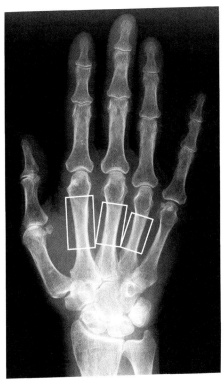

Fig. 3-31. X-ray image from computer-assisted radiogrammetry of the metacarpals of the index, long, and ring fingers. (Case provided courtesy of Pronosco, Denmark.)

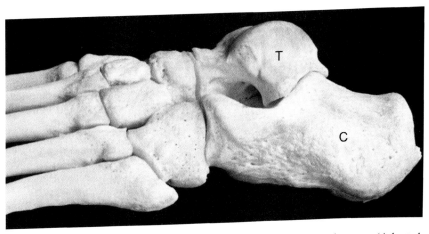

Fig. 3-32. Lateral view of the bones of the left foot. T, talus; C, calcaneus. (Adapted from McMinn, R. M. H., Hutchings, R. T., Pegington, J., et al. [1993] *Colour Atlas of Human Anatomy*, 3rd ed., p. 284. By permission of Mosby.)

C.C., Imhof, H. (1997) Impact of spinal degenerative changes on the evaluation of bone mineral density with dual energy X-ray absorptiometry (DXA). *Calcif. Tissue Int.* **60**, 430–433.

6. Cann, C. E., Rutt, B. K., Genant, H. K. (1983) Effect of extraosseous calcification on vertebral mineral measurement. *Calcif. Tissue Int.* **35**, 667.

7. Liu, G., Peacock, M., Eilam, O., Dorulla, G., Braunstein, E., Johnston, C.C. (1997) Effect of osteoarthritis in the lumbar spine and hip on bone mineral density and diagnosis of osteoporosis in elderly men and women. *Osteoporos. Int.* **7**, 564–569.

8. Frye, M. A., Melton, L. J., Bryant, S. C., Fitzpatrick, L. A., Wahner, H. W., Schwartz, R. S., Riggs, B. L. (1992) Osteoporosis and calcification of the aorta. *Bone Miner.* **19**, 185–194.

9. Frohn, J., Wilken, T., Falk, S., Stutte, H. J., Kollath, J., Hor, G. (1990) Effect of aortic sclerosis on bone mineral measurments by dual-photon absorptiometry. *J. Nucl. Med.* **32**, 259–262.

10. Orwoll, E. S., Oviatt, S. K., Mann, T. (1990) The impact of osteophytic and vascular calcifications on vertebral mineral density measurements in men. *J. Clin. Endocrinol. Metab.* **70**, 1202–1207.

11. Reid, I. R., Evans, M. C., Ames, R., Wattie, D. J. (1991) The influence of osteophytes and aortic calcification on spinal mineral density in post-menopausal women. *J. Clin. Endocrinol. Metab.* **72**, 1372–1374.

12. Banks, L. M., Lees, B., MacSweeney, J. E., Stevenson, J. C. (1991) Do degenerative changes and aortic calcification influence long-term bone density measurements? 8th International Workshop on Bone Densitometry, Bad Reichenhall, Germany.

13. Drinka, P. J., DeSmet, A. A., Bauwens, S. F., Rogot, A. (1992) The effect of overlying calcification on lumbar bone densitometry. *Calcif. Tissue Int.* **50**, 507–510.

14. Stutzman, M. E., Yester, M. V., Dubovsky, E. V. (1987) Technical aspects of dual-photon absorptiometry of the spine. *Technique* **15**, 177–181.

15. Rupich, R. C., Griffin, M. G., Pacifici, R., Avioli, L. V., Susman, N. (1992) Lateral dual-energy radiography: artifact error from rib and pelvic bone. *J. Bone Miner. Res.* **7**, 97–101.

16. Jergas, M., Breitenseher, M., Gluer, C. C., Black, D., Lang, P., Grampp, S., Engelke, K., Genant, H. K. (1995) Which vertebrae should be assessed using lateral dual-energy X-ray absorptiometry of the lumbar spine? *Osteoporos. Int.* **5**, 196–204.

17. Goh, J. C. H., Low, S. L., Bose, K. (1995) Effect of femoral rotation on bone mineral density measurements with dual energy X-ray absorptiometry. *Calcif. Tissue Int.* **57**, 340–343.

18. Bonnick, S. L., Nichols, D. L., Sanborn, C. F., Payne, S. G., Moen, S. M., Heiss, C. J. (1996) Right and left proximal femur analyses: is there a need to do both? *Calcif. Tissue Int.* **58**, 307–310.

19. Faulkner, K. G., Genant, H. K., McClung, M. (1995) Bilateral comparison of femoral bone density and hip axis length from single and fan beam DXA scans. *Calcif. Tissue Int.* **56**, 26–31.

20. Nevitt, M. C., Lane, N. E., Scott, J. C., Hochberg, M. C., Pressman, A. R., Genant, H. K., Cummings, S. R. (1995) Radiographic osteoarthritis of the hip and bone mineral density. *Arthritis Rheum.* **38**, 907–916.

21. Preidler, K. W., White, L. S., Tashkin, J., McDaniel, C. O., Brossman, J., Andresen, R., Sartoris, D. (1997) Dual-energy X-ray absorptiometric densitometry in osteoarthritis of the hip: influence of secondary bone remodeling of the femoral neck. *Acta Radiol.* **38**, 539–542.

22. Hans, D., Biot, B., Schott, A. M., Meunier, P. J. (1996) No diffuse osteoporosis in lumbar scoliosis but lower femoral bone density on the convexity. *Bone* **18,** 15–17.

23. Karjalainen, P. and Alhava, E. M. (1976) Bone mineral content of the forearm in a healthy population. *Acta Radiol. Oncol. Radiat. Phys. Biol.* **16,** 199–208.

24. Borg, J., Mollgaard, A., Riis, B. J. (1995) Single X-ray absorptiometry: performance characteristics and comparison with single photon absorptiometry. *Osteoporos. Int.* **5,** 377–381.

25. Huddleston, A. L., Rockwell, D., Kulund, D. N., Harrison, B. (1980) Bone mass in lifetime tennis athletes. *JAMA* **244,** 1107–1109.

26. Kannus, P., Haapasalo, H., Sievanen, H., Oja, P., Vuori, I. (1994) The site-specific effects of long-term unilateral activity on bone mineral density and content. *Bone* **15,** 279–284.

27. Akesson, K., Gardsell, P., Sernbo, I., Johnell, O., Obrant, K. J. (1992) Earlier wrist fracture: a confounding factor in distal forearm bone screening. *Osteoporos. Int.* **2,** 201–204.

28. Mussolino, M. E., Looker, A. C., Madans, J. H., Edelstein, D., Walker, R. E., Lydick, E., Epstein, R. S., Yates, A. J. (1997) Phalangeal bone density and hip fracture risk. *Arch. Intern. Med.* **157,** 433–438.

29. Huang, C., Ross, P. D., Yates, A. J., Walker, R. E., Imose, K., Emi, K., Wasnich, R. D. (1998) Prediction of fracture risk by radiographic absorptiometry and quantitative ultrasound: a prospective study. *Calcif. Tissue Int.* **6,** 380–384.

30. Cummings, S. R., Black, D. M., Nevitt, M. C., et al. (1993) Bone density at various sites for prediction of hip fractures. *Lancet* **341,** 72–75.

4 Densitometry Devices Approved by the Food and Drug Administration

CONTENTS

The devices discussed in this chapter are available in the United States for clinical use. The specifications were provided by the manufacturers and are subject to change without notice because devices are continually upgraded to reflect advances in the technology. The categories of information provided by each manufacturer may vary slightly. All categories are not relevant to every device. This listing of devices is not intended to reflect all devices in use in the United States. Every attempt was made to ensure the accuracy of the information. The manufacturer should be contacted for the latest specifications. The devices are grouped by type and listed alphabetically by model name.

COMPUTER-ENHANCED RADIOGRAMMETRY

Pronosco X-posure System™ 2.0 (Fig. 4-1)

- Manufacturer: Pronosco A/S, Denmark.
- Technique: Computerized radiogrammetry utilizing plain films of the hand. System consists of a Pentium III IBM-compatible computer with Windows NT™ and X-posure software installed, 15-in. color monitor, high-resolution X-ray image scanner, and color printer.

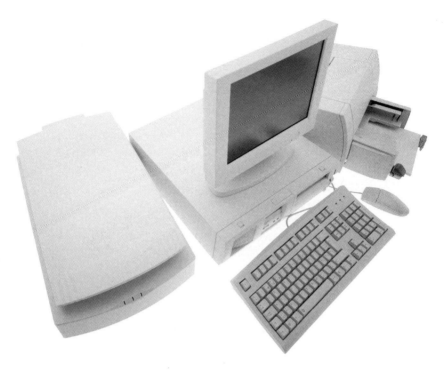

Fig. 4-1. Pronosco X-posure System. The system consists of the computer, monitor, mouse, printer, flatbed scanner, and analysis software to perform computer-assisted radiogrammetry. (Photograph courtesy of Pronosco, Denmark.)

- Skeletal applications: Metacarpals of the index, long, and ring fingers
- Results
    —BMD (g/cm^2).
    —Metacarpal index (MI).
    —% young adult and % age-matched comparisons.
    —T-score and z-score.
    —Fracture risk based on WHO classification.
- Patient scan time: Not applicable.
- Analysis time: <2 minutes for film scanning and analysis.
- Precision: 0.35%.
- Radiation exposure: 1 μSv limited to the hand during plain film acquisition.
- Quality control: Automated process to check for accuracy in film digitalization and placement of region of interest (ROI).
- Operation: A plain film of the hand is acquired. Patient data are entered from the computer keyboard. The plain film of the hand is

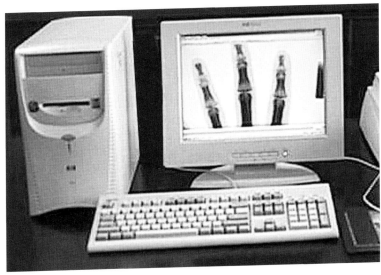

Fig. 4-2. CompuMed Automated Osteogram Analysis System. The system consists of the computer, monitor, mouse, flatbed scanner, and analysis software to perform computer-assisted radiographic photodensitometry of the phalanges. (Photograph courtesy of CompuMed, Los Angeles, CA.)

digitized by scanning the film. The X-posure software automatically places the ROIs and calculates the BMD and MI. The system is designed to integrate with future digital X-ray capture technologies and computer networks.

COMPUTER-ENHANCED RADIOGRAPHIC ABSORPTIOMETRY

Automated OsteoGram® (Fig. 4-2)

- Manufacturer: CompuMed, Los Angeles, CA.
- Technique: Radiographic absorptiometry (RA) utilizing plain films of the hand with a computerized analysis. The system consists of an HP® minitower computer with OsteoGram® software installed, 15-in. flat panel display monitor, AGFA DuoScan T1200 scanner, keyboard, and mouse.
- Skeletal applications: Middle phalanges of the index, long, and middle fingers.

- Results
  —BMD in arbitrary RA units.
  —T-score and z-score.
  —Diagnostic classification based on WHO criteria.
- Patient scan time: Not applicable.
- Analysis time: Approximately 1 minute, excluding film digitization time
- Precision: <1%.
- Quality control: Automated system checks to ensure quality and accuracy of image digitalization.
- Operation: Two hand films are taken. Data are entered into the computer program with the computer keyboard. The plain film is scanned into the computer and then analyzed by proprietary software installed on the computer. The results are then printed.
- Accessories provided
  —SCSI interface connector.
  —CMI/AGFA Ortho 400 Green Cassette with the OsteoGram film template mounted with the reference wedge.
  —Mouse pad.
  —Clinical Overview CD.
  —Procedure video.
  —Instruction manual.

MetriScan™ (Fig. 4-3)

- Manufacturer: Alara, Hayward, CA.
- Technique: Radiographic absorptiometry (RA) with storage phosphor technology.
- Skeletal applications: Middle phalanges of the index, long, and ring fingers.
- Scan time: 1 second.
- Results
  —Estimated phalangeal BMD in arbitrary RA units.
  —% Young adult and % age-matched comparisons.
  —T-score and z-score.
  —Diagnostic classification based on WHO criteria.
- Precision: 1.1%.
- Radiation exposure: 0.0001 mrem/scan (0.001 μSv/scan).
- Dimensions: 16 in. × 16 in. × 16 in. (40.6 cm × 40.6 cm × 40.6 cm).
- Weight: 41.5 lb (18.8 kg).
- Environmental operating temperature: 64° F to 95° F (18° to 35° C).
- Environmental operating humidity: 5%–80%, noncondensing.

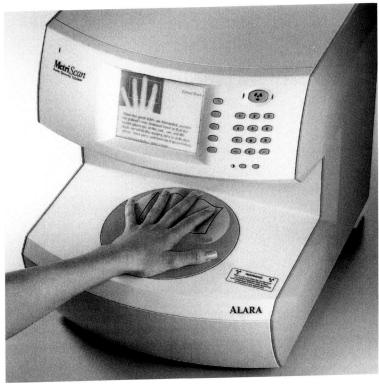

Fig. 4-3. Alara MetriScan. This is a self-contained X-ray unit used to perform radiographic absorptiometry of the phalanges. (Photograph courtesy of Alara, Hayward, CA.)

- Scatter radiation: 0.0001 mrem/scan (0.001 μSv/scan) at 1 m.
- Quality control: Automated.
- Operation: The unit is self-contained and does not require a standard hand film. Data are input from the keypad on the unit. A separate HP DeskJet 697C or 710C printer or printer as specified by Alara is needed for results output.

CENTRAL X-RAY DENSITOMETERS

Delphi™ (Fig. 4-4)

- Manufacturer: Hologic, Bedford, MA.
- Technology: Dual energy X-ray absorptiometry (DXA).

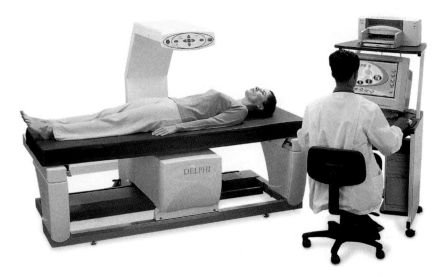

Fig. 4-4. Hologic Delphi. This is a central fan-array dual-energy X-ray absorptiometer. (Photograph courtesy of Hologic, Bedford, MA.)

- Skeletal applications
  —PA lumbar spine.
  —Proximal femur.
  —Forearm.
  —IVA™ lateral spine imaging (T4–L4).
  —Dual Hip™
  —Whole body: (on Delphi™ with Whole Body).
- Scan time (in 60-Hz scan mode)
  —PA lumbar spine and proximal femur: 15 seconds.
  —Forearm: 30 seconds.
  —Whole body: 6.8 minutes.
  —Single energy IVA: 10 seconds (for 15-in. scan length).
- Results
  —BMD (g/cm^2).
  —BMC (g).
  —Area (cm^2).
  —T-score and z-score.
  —sBMD (mg/cm^2).
  —NHANES III reference data for hip.
  —Trend reports for serial monitoring.

- Precision: <1.0%.
- Radiation dose (in 60-Hz scan mode)
  —PA lumbar spine and proximal femur: 5 mR.
  —Forearm: 10 mR.
  —Whole body: 1.5 mR.
  —IVA: 7 mR (15-in. scan length).
- Dimensions
  —Delphi 76 × 49.5 × 28 in. (193 × 126 × 71 cm).
  —Delphi with Whole Body: 79.5 × 48 × 28 in. (202 × 122 × 71 cm), 119 × 59 × 28 in. (302 × 150 × 71 cm) table extended.
- Weight
  —Delphi 650 lb (296 kg).
  —Delphi with Whole Body: 680 lb (310 kg).
- Recommended dedicated floor space: 8 × 8 ft (2.4 × 2.4 m).
- Scatter radiation: 1.0 mR/hr (0.01 mSv/hour) measured at 2.0 m (6.6 ft) from the examination table for most scan modes.
- Operating environmental temperature: 15° to 32°C (60° to 90°F)
- Operating environmental relative humidity: 20% to 80%, noncondensing.
- X-ray source: Switched pulse at 140 kVp and 100 kVp for dual energy; 140 kVp for single energy IVA.
- X-ray beam geometry: Fan.
- Detectors: Multielement detector array.
- Scan path: Linear.
- Quality control: Self-calibrating with Hologic Automatic Internal Reference system and automated quality control program.
- Operation: IBM-compatible Pentium™ computer, Windows 98®-based operating system, HP DeskJet® printer, 17-in. monitor.
- Accessories provided
  —Anthropomorphic spine phantom.
  —Medical imaging printer.
- Options: Magneto-optical disk storage; HP LaserJet® black-and-white printer; flat panel monitor; whole body, body composition analysis, and quantitative morphometry software; modem or network options.

DPX-IQ™ (Fig. 4-5)

- Manufacturer: GE Lunar, Madison, WI.
- Technology: Dual energy X-ray absorptiometry.

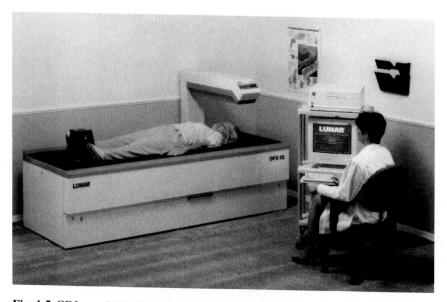

Fig. 4-5. GE Lunar DPX-IQ. This is a central pencil-beam dual-energy X-ray absorptiometer. (Photograph courtesy of GE Lunar, Madison, WI.)

- Skeletal applications
  —PA spine.
  —Proximal femur.
  —Total body with soft-tissue quantification (only with full-size table).
- Scan time
  —PA spine: 2 minutes.
  —Proximal femur: 2 minutes.
  —Total body: 11 minutes.
- Results
  —BMD (g/cm²).
  —BMC (g).
  —Area (cm²).
  —% Young adult and % age-matched comparisons.
  —T-score, z-score.
  —sBMD (mg/cm²) for L2–L4 and total hip.
  —NHANES III total hip comparisons.
- Precision
  —PA spine: 0.5%.
  —Hip: 1%.

—Total body: 0.5%.
- Radiation dose
  —PA spine or proximal femur: <3 mrem.
  —Total body: 0.02 mrem.
- Dimensions
  —Full-size table: 95 × 42 × 52 in. (242 × 107 × 133 cm).
  —Compact table: 71 × 40 × 52 in. (181 × 100 × 133 cm).
- Weight
  —Full-size table: 598 lb (272 kg).
  —Compact table: 550 lb (250 kg).
- Recommended dedicated floor space
  —Full-size table: 9 × 7 ft (2 × 2.1 m).
  —Compact table: 7 × 7 ft (2.1 × 2.1 m).
- Operating environmental temperature: 65–80° F (18–27° C).
- Operating environmental relative humidity: 30–75%, noncondensing.
- X-ray source: 134 kVp; 3.0 mA for PA spine and proximal femur studies (milliamperes vary by skeletal site and scan mode).
- X-ray filtration: constant potential, cerium K-edge filter.
- X-ray beam geometry: Pencil.
- Detectors: NaI.
- Scan path: Rectilinear.
- Quality control: Block phantom and aluminum spine phantom supplied by manufacturer.
- Operation: IBM-compatible desktop Pentium computer, SVGA monitor, printer.
- Accessories provided
  —PA spine-positioning block.
  —Foot positioner for proximal femur studies.
  —Block phantom.
  —Aluminum spine phantom.
- Options: Forearm, hand, lateral spine, and orthopedics software; forearm positioner; lateral spine positioner; encapsulated spine phantom.

DPX MD™

- Manufacturer: GE Lunar, Madison, WI.
- Technology: Dual energy X ray absorptiometry.
- Skeletal applications
  —PA spine.
  —Proximal femur.

—DualFemur™ (not available on compact model).
—Total body (not available on compact model).
- Scan time
  —PA spine and proximal femur: 2 minutes.
  —DualFemur: 4 minutes.
  —Total body: 8 minutes.
- Results
  —BMD (g/cm^2).
  —BMC (g).
  —% young adult and % age-matched comparisons.
  —T-score, z-score.
  —sBMD (mg/cm^2).
  —NHANES III reference data.
  —WHO diagnostic classification.
- Precision
  —PA spine and total femur: 1.0%.
  —DualFemur: 0.7%.
  —Total body: 0.5%.
- Radiation dose
  —PA spine: 1 mrem.
  —Femur: 1 mrem.
  —Total body: 0.02 mrem.
- Dimensions
  —Full-size table: 95 × 42 × 52 in. (242 × 107 × 133 cm).
  —Compact table: 71 × 40 × 52 in. (181 × 100 × 133 cm).
- Weight
  —Full-size table: 598 lb (272 kg).
  —Compact table: 550 lb (250 kg).
- Recommended dedicated floor space
  —Full-size table: 9 × 7 ft (2.7 × 2.1 m).
  —Compact table: 7 × 7 ft (2.1 × 2.1 m).
- Operating environmental temperature: 65–80° F (18–27° C).
- Operating environmental relative humidity: 30% to 75%, noncondensing.
- X-ray source: 134 kV; 0.75 mA for PA spine, proximal femur, DualFemur (mA varies by skeletal site and scan mode).
- X-ray filtration: Constant potential, cerium K-edge filter.
- X-ray beam geometry: Pencil.
- Detectors: NaI.
- Scan path: Rectilinear.
- Quality control: Automatic test program.

- Operation: IBM-compatible computer, printer.
- Accessories provided
  —PA spine positioner.
  —Proximal femur positioner.
  —DualFemur positioner.
  —Aluminum spine phantom.
- Options: Lateral spine, forearm/hand, pediatrics, orthopedics, and small animal software; encapsulated phantom.

DPX MD+™

- Manufacturer: GE Lunar, Madison, WI.
- Technology: Dual energy X ray absorptiometry.
- Skeletal applications
  —PA spine.
  —Proximal femur.
- Results
  —BMD (g/cm^2).
  —BMC (g).
  —% Young adult and % age-matched comparisons.
  —T-score and z-score.
  —sBMD (mg/cm^2).
  —NHANES III reference data.
  —WHO diagnostic classification.
- Precision
  —PA spine, proximal femur, and total body: 1.0%.
  —DualFemur: <1.0%.
- Radiation dose
  —PA spine and proximal femur: 3.0 mrem.
  —Total body: 0.02 mrem.
- Dimensions
  —Full-size table: 95 × 42 × 52 in. (242 × 107 × 133 cm).
  —Compact table: 71 × 40 × 52 in. (181 × 100 × 133 cm).
- Weight
  —Full-size table: 598 lb (272 kg).
  —Compact table: 550 lb (250 kg).
- Recommended dedicated floor space
  —Full-size table: 9 × 7 ft (2.7 × 2.1 m).
  —Compact table: 7 × 7 ft (2.1 × 2.1 m).
- Operating environmental temperature: 65–80° F (18–27° C).
- Operating environmental relative humidity: 30% to 75%, noncondensing.

- X-ray source: 134 kV; 0.75 mA for PA spine, proximal femur, DualFemur.
- X-ray filtration: Constant potential, cerium K-edge filter.
- X-ray beam geometry: Pencil.
- Detectors: NaI.
- Scan path: Rectilinear.
- Quality control: Automatic test program.
- Operation: IBM-compatible computer, printer.
- Accessories provided
  —PA spine positioner.
  —Proximal femur positioner.
  —Aluminum spine phantom.
- Options: DualFemur with positioner (not available on compact model), total body with body composition (not available on compact model); encapsulated phantom.

DPX-NT™

- Manufacturer: GE Lunar Madison, WI.
- Technology: Dual energy X ray absorptiometry
- Skeletal applications
  —PA spine.
  —Proximal femur.
  —DualFemur.
  —Total body with body composition.
- Scan time
  —PA spine: 1 minute.
  —Proximal femur: 2 minutes.
  —DualFemur: 4 minutes.
  —Total body: 8 minutes.
- Results
  —BMD (g/cm^2).
  —sBMD (mg/cm^2).
  —T-score and z-score.
  —NHANES III reference data.
  —WHO diagnostic classification.
- Precision
  —PA spine: 1.0%.
  —Proximal femur: 1.0%.
  —Total body: 1.0%.
  —DualFemur: <1.0%.

- Radiation dose
  —PA spine: 3.0 mrem.
  —Proximal femur: 3.0 mrem.
  —Total body: 0.02 mrem.
- Dimensions: 95 × 42 × 52 in. (242 × 107 × 133 cm).
- Weight: 598 lb (272 kg).
- Recommended dedicated floor space: 9 × 7 ft (2.7 × 2.1 m).
- Operating environmental temperature: 65–80° F (18–27° C).
- Operating environmental relative humidity: 30% to 75%, noncondensing.
- X-ray source: 134 kV; 1.5 mA for PA spine, proximal femur, Dual-Femur (mA varies by skeletal site and scan mode).
- X-ray filtration: Constant potential, cerium K-edge filter.
- X-ray beam geometry: Pencil.
- Detectors: NaI.
- Scan path: Rectilinear.
- Quality control: Automated QA program.
- Operation: IBM-compatible computer running Windows NT.
- Accessories provided
  —PA spine positioner.
  —Proximal femur positioner.
  —DualFemur positioner.
  —Aluminum spine phantom.
- Options: Encapsulated phantom.

Excell™ (Fig. 4-6)

- Manufacturer: Norland Medical Systems, Ft. Atkinson, WI.
- Technology: Dual energy X-ray absorptiometry.
- Standard application(s)
  —PA spine.
  —Proximal femur.
- Scan time
  —PA spine: <1.5 minutes.
  —Proximal femur: <2 minutes.
- Results
  —BMD (g/cm^2).
  —BMC (g).
  —Length (cm).
  —% young reference and % age-matched comparisons.
  —T-score and z-score.
  —sBMD (mg/cm^2) for L2–L4 and total hip.

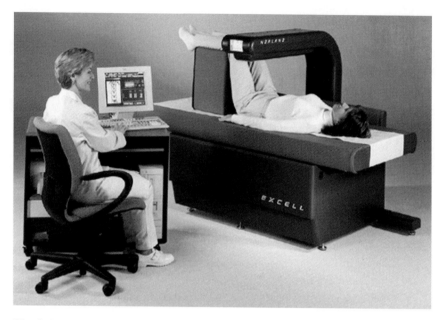

Fig. 4-6. Norland Excell. This is a central pencil-beam X-ray absorptiometer. (Photograph courtesy of Norland Medical Systems, Ft. Atkinson, WI.)

—NHANES III total hip comparisons.
—Fracture risk based on WHO diagnostic classification.
- Precision
  —PA spine: 1.0%.
  —Hip: 1.2%.
- Radiation dose: <1.0 mrem in high-speed scan mode.
- Dimensions: 72 × 48 × 49 in. (182.8 × 122.0 × 124.5 cm).
- Weight: 400 lb (181 kg).
- Recommended dedicated floor space: 7 × 7 ft (2.1 × 2.1 m).
- Operating environmental temperature: 60–104° F (15–40° C).
- Operating environmental relative humidity: up to 80%, noncondensing.
- X-ray source: 100 kV, 1.3 mA.
- X-ray filtration: Samarium.
- X-ray beam geometry: Pencil beam.
- Detectors: Two NaI scintillation detectors.
- Scan path: Rectilinear.
- Quality control: Automated with 77-step calibration standard and quality control phantom.

- Operation: IBM-compatible PC computer, HP DeskJet.
- Accessories provided
  —PA spine-positioning block.
  —Hip sling with foot separator.
  —77-Step calibration standard.
  —Quality control phantom.
- Options: Laptop computer.

Excell™plus

- Manufacturer: Norland Medical Systems, Ft. Atkinson, WI.
- Technology: Dual energy X-ray absorptiometry.
- Skeletal applications
  —PA spine.
  —Proximal femur.
  —Forearm.
  —Lateral spine.
- Scan time
  —PA spine: <1.5 minutes.
  —Proximal femur: <2 minutes.
  —Forearm: <3 minutes.
  —Lateral spine: <4 minutes.
- Results
  —BMD (g/cm^2).
  —BMC (g).
  —Length (cm).
  —% young reference and % age-matched comparisons.
  —T-score, z-score.
  —sBMD (mg/cm^2) for L2–L4 and total hip.
  —NHANES III total hip comparisons.
- Precision
  —PA spine: 1.0%.
  —Hip: 1.2%.
  —Forearm: 0.8%.
  —Lateral spine: 2.4%.
- Radiation dose
  —PA spine, proximal femur, forearm: <1.0 mrem.
  —Lateral spine: <2 mrem.
- Dimensions: 72 × 48 × 49 in. (182.8 × 122.0 × 124.5 cm).
- Weight: 400 lb (181 kg).
- Recommended dedicated floor space: 7 × 7 ft (2.1 × 2.1 m).
- Operating environmental temperature: 60–104° F (15–40° C).

- Operating environmental relative humidity: up to 80%, noncondensing.
- X-ray source: 100 kV, 1.3 mA.
- X-ray filtration: Samarium.
- X-ray beam geometry: Pencil.
- Detectors: Two NaI scintillation detectors.
- Scan path: Rectilinear.
- Quality control: Automated with 77-step calibration standard and quality control phantom.
- Operation: IBM-compatible computer with Windows operating system, DeskJet printer, 15-in. SVGA monitor.
- Accessories provided
  —PA spine-positioning block.
  —Hip sling with foot separator for use in proximal femur studies.
  —Lateral and forearm positioning aids.
  —77-Step calibration standard.
  —Quality control phantom.
- Options: Software for research, small subject, or body composition; laptop computer; flat-screen monitor; 17-in. SVGA monitor.

EXPERT®-XL (Fig. 4-7)

- Manufacturer: GE Lunar, Madison, WI.
- Technology: Dual energy X-ray absorptiometry.
- Skeletal applications
  —PA spine.
  —Lateral lumbar spine.
  —Proximal femur.
  —Forearm and hand.
  —Total body.
  —Orthopedic hip.
  —Vertebral morphometry.
- Scan times
  —PA spine and proximal femur: 6 seconds.
  —Forearm/hand: 10 seconds.
  —Lateral spine: 24 seconds.
  —Total body: 160 seconds.
  —Vertebral morphometry: 38 seconds.
- Results
  —BMD (g/cm^2).
  —BMC (g).
  —Area (cm^2).

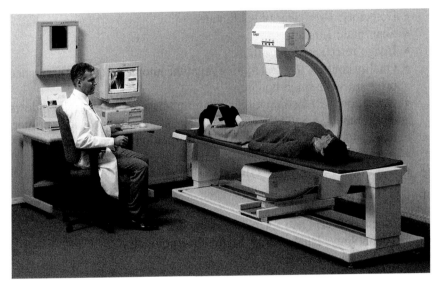

Fig. 4-7. GE Lunar Expert-XL. This is a central fan-array dual-energy X-ray absorptiometer. (Photograph courtesy of GE Lunar, Madison, WI.)

—% young adult and % age-matched comparsions.
—T-score and z-score.
—Vertebral heights (mm) and vertebral height ratios.
- Precision: 1.0%.
- Radiation dose
  —PA spine and proximal femur: 27 mrem.
  —Forearm/hand: 12 mrem.
  —Lateral spine: 190 mrem.
  —Total body: 5 mrem.
  —Morphometry: 120 mrem.
- Dimensions: 108 × 71 in. (2.7 × 1.8 m). Motorized C-arm 140° rotation with 78-in. (198-cm) longitudinal travel and 14-in. (36-cm) transverse travel.
- Weight: 750 lb (340.2 kg).
- Recommended dedicated floor space: 12 × 10 ft (3.7 × 3.1 m).
- Operating environmental temperature: 65–80° F (18–27° C).
- Operating environmental relative humidity: 30 to 75%, noncondensing.
- X-ray source: 134 kV; 5 mA for PA spine, proximal femur, lateral spine, and morphometry.
- X-ray beam geometry: Fan beam.

- Detectors: Dual energy solid state.
- Scan path: Linear.
- Image resolution: 0.5 mm.
- Quality control: Internal hydroxyapatite; automated quality assurance program with spine phantom.
- Operation: IBM-compatible, Pentium®-based computer; Windows environment; SVGA monitor; black-and-white laser printer; handheld motor controller for C-arm rotation and table elevation.
- Accessories provided: Spine phantom.
- Options: Color printer, DICOM utilities.

Prodigy™ (Fig. 4-8)

- Manufacturer: GE Lunar, Madison, WI.
- Technology: Dual energy X-ray absorptiometry
- Skeletal applications
  —PA spine.
  —Proximal femur.
  —DualFemur.
  —Customized ROI with metal removal.
  —Total body and body composition.
- Scan time
  —PA spine and proximal femur: 30 seconds.
  —DualFemur: 1 minute.
  —Total body: 5 minutes.
- Results
  —BMD (g/cm^2).
  —sBMD (mg/cm^2).
  —T-score, z-score.
  —Fracture risk assessment based on WHO diagnostic classification.
  —LUNAR® and NHANES III databases.
- Precision
  —PA spine and proximal femur: 1.0%.
  —DualFemur: <1.0%.
  —Total body: <1.0%.
- Radiation dose
  —PA spine and proximal femur: 3.7 mrem.
  —Total body: 0.037 mrem.
- Dimensions: 103.5 × 43.5 × 50 in. (263 × 111 × 127 cm).
- Weight: 600 lb (272 kg).
- Recommended dedicated floor space: 9 × 7.5 ft (2.8 × 2.3 m).
- Scatter radiation: <0.3 mrad/hour (3 µSv/hour) at 39 in. (1 m).

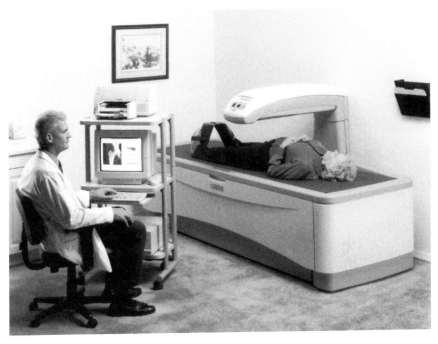

Fig. 4-8. GE Lunar Prodigy. This is a central fan-array dual-energy X-ray absorptiometer. (Photograph courtesy of GE Lunar, Madison, WI.)

- Operating environmental temperature: 65–80° F (18–27° C).
- Operating environmental relative humidity: 20 to 80%, noncondensing.
- X-ray source: 134 kV; 3.0 mA for PA spine, proximal femur, Lateral Vertebral Assessment (milliamperes vary by skeletal site and scan mode).
- X-ray filtration: Constant potential, cerium K-edge filter.
- X-ray beam geometry: Narrow-angle fan.
- Detectors: Cadium-zinc-telluride.
- Scan path: Rectilinear.
- Quality control: Automatic test program with QA trending.
- Operation: Windows NT–based program on IBM-compatible Pentium computer, printer.
- Accessories provided
  —PA spine positioner.
  —DualFemur positioner.
  —Aluminum spine phantom.

- Options: Pediatric, forearm, lateral spine, and LateralView™ software; encapsulated phantom.

QDR® 4500 A   (Figs. 4-9 and 4-10)

- Manufacturer: Hologic, Bedford, MA.
- Technology: Dual energy X-ray absorptiometry.
- Skeletal applications
  —PA spine.
  —Proximal femur.
  —Forearm.
  —Whole body.
  —Supine lateral lumbar spine.
- Scan time (in 60-Hz scan mode).
  —PA lumbar spine and proximal femur: 10 seconds.
  —Lateral spine: 120 seconds.
  —Forearm: 30 seconds.
  —Whole body: 3 minutes.
  —Lateral imaging with MXA: 7.5 seconds.
- Results
  —BMD (g/cm^2).
  —BMC (g).
  —Area (cm^2).
  —% Young adult and % age-matched comparisons.
  —T-score and z-score.
  —sBMD (mg/cm^2) for L2–L4 and total hip.
  —NHANES III total hip comparisons.
- Precision: <1%.
- Radiation dose (in 60-Hz scan mode)
  —PA lumbar: 7 mR.
  —Proximal femur: 7 mR.
  —Lateral spine: 35 mR.
  —Forearm: 5 mR.
  —Whole body: 1 mR.
  —Lateral imaging with MXA: 7 mR.
- Dimensions: 79.5 × 41 × 28 in. (202 × 104 × 71 cm), 118.9 × 57 in. (302 × 145 cm) with c-arm rotated and table extended.
- Weight: 800 lb (364 kg).
- Recommended dedicated floor space: 8 × 10 ft (2.4 × 3.1 m).
- Scatter radiation: Less than 1.0 mR/hr (0.01 mSv/hour) measured at 6.6 ft (2.0 m) from the examination table for most scan modes.
- Operating environmental temperature: 60–90° F (15–32° C).

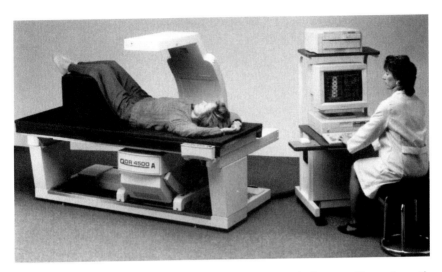

Fig. 4-9. Hologic QDR 4500 A. This is a central fan-array dual-energy X-ray absorptiometer. (Photo courtesy of Hologic, Bedford, MA.)

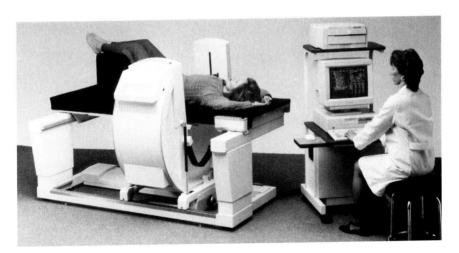

Fig. 4-10. Hologic QDR 4500 A. The gantry is rotated to perform supine lateral lumbar spine studies. (Photograph courtesy of Hologic, Bedford, MA.)

- Operating environmental relative humidity: 20 to 80%.
- X-ray source: Switched pulse, dual energy.
- X-ray beam geometry: Fan.
- Detectors: Multielement detector array.
- Scan path: Linear.

- Quality control: Self-calibrating with patented Hologic Automatic Internal Reference System and automated quality control program.
- Operation: IBM-compatible Pentium computer with Windows operating system, 17-in. monitor, HP LaserJet black-and-white printer.
- Accessories provided: Anthropomorphic spine phantom.
- Options: Magneto-optical disk storage; network configurations; body composition analysis software, MXA software, small animal software.

QDR® 4500 C

- Manufacturer: Hologic, Bedford, MA.
- Technology: Dual energy X-ray absorptiometry.
- Skeletal applications
  —PA spine.
  —Proximal femur.
  —Forearm.
- Scan time (in 60-Hz scan mode)
  —PA lumbar spine and proximal femur: 15 seconds.
  —Forearm: 30 seconds.
- Results
  —BMD (g/cm^2).
  —BMC (g).
  —Area (cm^2).
  —% Young adult and % age-matched comparisons.
  —T-score and z-score.
  — sBMD (mg/cm^2) for L2–L4 and total hip.
  —NHANES III total hip comparisons.
  —Fracture risk and diagnostic classification based on WHO criteria.
- Precision: <1%.
- Radiation dose (in 60-Hz scan mode)
  —PA lumbar spine: 5 mR.
  —Proximal femur: 5 mR.
  —Forearm: 10 mR.
- Dimensions: 79.5 × 41 × 28 in. (202 × 104 × 71 cm).
- Weight: 650 lb (296 kg).
- Recommended dedicated floor space: 8 × 8 ft (2.4 × 2.4 m).
- Scatter radiation: Less than 1.0 mrad/hour (0.01 mSv/hour) measured at 6.6 ft (2.0 m) from the examination table for most scan modes.
- Operating environmental temperature: 60–90° F (15–32° C).

- Operating environmental relative humidity: 20% to 80%, noncondensing.
- X-ray source: Switched pulse, dual energy, 140-V peak.
- X-ray beam geometry: Fan.
- Detectors: Multielement detector array.
- Scan path: Linear.
- Quality control: Self-calibrating with patented Hologic Automatic Internal Reference System and automated quality control program.
- Operation: IBM-compatible Pentium computer with Windows operating system, 17-in. monitor, HP DeskJet printer.
- Accessories provided: Anthropomorphic spine phantom.
- Options: Magneto-optical disk storage; network configuration; HP LaserJet black-and-white printer.

QDR® 4500 SL

- Manufacturer: Hologic, Bedford, MA.
- Technology: Dual energy X-ray absorptiometry.
- Skeletal applications
    —PA spine.
    —Proximal femur.
    —Forearm.
    —Supine lateral lumbar spine.
- Scan time (in 60-Hz scan mode)
    —PA lumbar spine and proximal femur: 10 seconds.
    —Lateral spine: 120 seconds.
    —Forearm: 30 seconds.
    —Lateral imaging with MXA: 7.5 seconds.
- Results
    —BMD (g/cm^2).
    —BMC (g).
    —Area (cm^2).
    —% Young adult and % age-matched comparisons.
    —T-score and z-score.
    — sBMD (mg/cm^2) for L2–L4 and total hip.
    —NHANES III total hip comparisons.
- Precision: <1%.
- Radiation dose (in 60-Hz scan mode)
    —PA lumbar spine: 7 mR.
    —Proximal femur: 7 mR.
    —Lateral spine: 35 mR.

—Forearm: 5 mR.

—Lateral imaging with MXA: 7 mR.

- Dimensions: 79.5 × 41 × 28 in. (202 × 104 × 71 cm), 79.5 × 57 in. (202 × 145 cm) with c-arm rotated and table extended.
- Weight: 800 lb (364 kg).
- Recommended dedicated floor space: 8 × 8 ft (2.4 × 2.4 m).
- Scatter radiation: Less than 1.0 mR/hr (0.01 mSv/hour) measured at 6.6 ft (2.0 m) from the examination table for most scan modes.
- Operating environmental temperature: 60–90° F (15–32° C).
- Operating environmental relative humidity: 20% to 80%.
- X-ray source: Switched pulse, dual energy.
- X-ray beam geometry: Fan.
- Detectors: Multielement detector array.
- Scan path: Linear.
- Quality control: Self-calibrating with patented Hologic Automatic Internal Reference System and automated quality control program.
- Operation: IBM-compatible Pentium computer with Windows operating system, 17-in. monitor, HP DeskJet printer.
- Accessories provided: Anthropomorphic spine phantom.
- Options: Magneto-optical disk storage; network configurations; HP LaserJet black-and-white printer; MXA software.

QDR® 4500 W

- Manufacturer: Hologic, Bedford, MA.
- Technology: Dual energy X-ray absoprtiometry.
- Skeletal regions studied
  —PA spine.
  —Proximal femur.
  —Forearm.
  —Whole body.
- Scan time (in 60-Hz scan mode)
  —PA lumbar spine and proximal femur: 15 seconds.
  —Forearm: 30 seconds.
  —Whole body: 6.8 minutes.
- Results
  —BMD (g/cm^2).
  —BMC (g).
  —Area (cm^2).
  —% Young adult and % age-matched comparisons.
  —T-score and z-score.
  —sBMD (mg/cm^2) for L2–L4 and total hip.

—NHANES III total hip comparisons.
- Precision: <1%.
- Radiation dose (in 60-Hz scan mode).
  —PA lumbar spine: 5 mR.
  —Proximal femur: 5 mR.
  —Forearm: 10 mR.
  —Whole body: 1.5 mR.
- Dimensions: 79.5 × 48 × 28 in. (202 × 122 × 71 cm), 118.9 × 59 × 28 in. (302 × 150 × 71 cm) with table extended.
- Weight: 680 lb (310 kg).
- Recommended dedicated floor space: 8 × 10 ft (2.4 × 3.1 m).
- Scatter radiation: Less than 1.0 mR/hr (<0.01 mSv/hour) measured at 6.6 ft (2.0 m) from the examination table for most scan modes.
- Operating environmental temperature: 60–90° F (15–32° C).
- Operating environmental relative humidity: 20% to 80%.
- X-ray source: Switched pulse, dual energy.
- X-ray beam geometry: Fan.
- Detectors: Multielement detector array.
- Scan path: Linear.
- Quality control: Self-calibrating with patented Hologic Automatic Internal Reference System and automated quality control program.
- Operation: IBM-compatible Pentium computer with Windows operating system, 17-in. monitor, HP DeskJet printer.
- Accessories provided: Anthropomorphic spine phantom.
- Options: Magneto-optical disk storage; network configurations; HP LaserJet black-and-white printer; body composition analysis software.

XR-46™ (Fig. 4-11)

- Manufacturer: Norland Medical Systems, Ft. Atkinson, WI.
- Technology: Dual energy X-ray absorptiometry.
- Skeletal regions studied
  —PA spine.
  —Lateral spine.
  —Proximal femur.
  —Forearm.
  —Whole body with soft-tissue composition.
- Scan time
  —PA spine: <1.5 minutes.
  —Hip: <2 minutes.
  —Forearm: <3 minutes.

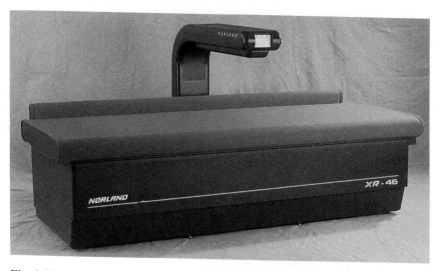

Fig. 4-11. Norland XR-46. This is a central pencil-beam dual-energy X-ray absorptiometer. (Photograph courtesy of Norland Medical Systems, Ft. Atkinson, WI.)

    —Lateral spine: <4 minutes.
    —Whole body: 5 minutes.
- Results
    —BMD (g/cm^2).
    —BMC (g).
    —% Young-reference and % age-matched comparisons.
    —T-score and z-score.
    —sBMD (mg/cm^2) for L2–L4 and total hip based on NHANES III
      reference data.
- Precision
    —PA spine: 1.0%.
    —Hip: 1.2%.
    —Forearm: 0.8%.
    —Lateral Spine: 2.4%.
    —Whole-body BMD: 1%.
- Radiation dose
    —PA spine, hip and forearm: <1.0 mrem.
    —Lateral spine: <5 mrem.
    —Whole body: <0.1 mrem.
- Dimensions: 103 × 48 × 51 in. (261.6 × 122.0 × 129.5 cm).
- Weight: 556.5 lbs (252.4 kg).
- Recommended dedicated floor space: 10 × 7 ft (3.1 × 2.1 m).

- Operating environmental temperatures: 60–90° F (15–32° C).
- Operating environmental relative humidity: Up to 80%, noncondensing.
- X-ray source: 100 kV, 1.3 mA.
- X-ray filtration: eight-level automated samarium.
- X-ray beam geometry: Pencil.
- Detectors: Two NaI detectors.
- Scan path: Rectilinear.
- Quality control: Automatic with supplied calibration standard and QC phantom.
- Operation: IBM-compatible computer with HP color DeskJet printer; DOS program with Microsoft Windows™ resident.
- Accessories provided
  —77-Step calibration standard.
  —QC phantom.
  —PA spine-positioning block.
  —Hip sling with foot separator.
  —Lateral spine positioner.
  —Forearm positioner.
- Options: Flat panel display 17-in. SVGA monitor, laptop configuration, Research and Small Subject software.

PERIPHERAL X-RAY DENSITOMETERS

accuDEXA™ (Fig. 4-12)

- Manufacturer: Schick Technologies, Long Island City, NY.
- Technology: DXA.
- Skeletal applications: Middle phalanx of the long finger.
- Scan time: <1 minute.
- Results
  —BMD (g/cm^2).
  —% Young adult and % age-matched comparisons.
  —T-score and z-score.
  —Diagnostic classification based on WHO criteria.
- Precision: <1%.
- Radiation dose: 0.0003 μSv.
- Dimensions: 14 × 15 × 14 in. (35.56 × 38.1 × 35.56 cm).
- Weight: 66 lbs (29.7 kg).
- Environmental operating temperature: 70–85° F (21–29° C).

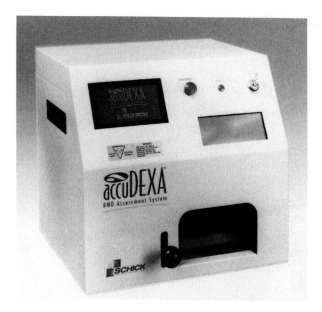

Fig. 4-12. Schick accuDEXA. This is a peripheral dual-energy X-ray absorptiometer used to measure bone density in the phalanges. (Photograph courtesy of Schick Technologies, Long Island City, NY.)

- Environmental operating relative humidity: 20% to 80%.
- X-ray source
  —Low energy: 50 kVp, 0.5 mA.
  —High energy: 70 kVp, 0.9 mA.
- X-ray filtration (only high energy): Zinc.
- Scatter radiation: 6.1 mR/hr at 1 m.
- Quality control: Automatic, no user intervention required.
- Operation: Data input with touch pad on the device, data output with printer supplied by user (list of compatible printers available from manufacturer).

Apollo™ (Fig. 4-13)

- Norland Medical Systems, Ft. Atkinson, WI.
- Technology: Dual-energy X-ray absorptiometry.
- Skeletal applications: Calcaneus.
- Scan time: 15 seconds.
- Results
  —BMD (g/cm^2).
  —BMC (g).

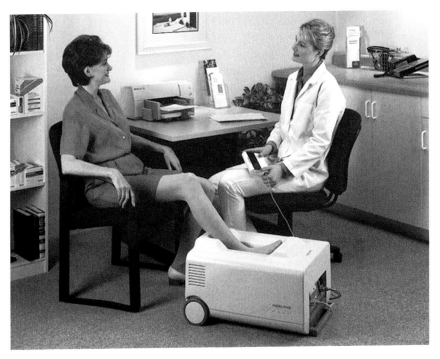

Fig. 4-13. Norland Apollo. This is a peripheral dual-energy X-ray absorptiometer used to measured bone density in the calcaneus. (Photograph courtesy of Norland Medical Systems, Ft. Atkinson, WI.)

—Area (cm^2).
—% Young reference and % age-matched comparisons.
—T-score and z-score.
—Fracture risk based on WHO diagnostic classification.
- Precision: 1.8%.
- Radiation dose: <0.2 mrem.
- Dimensions: 22.5 × 17.5 × 14 in. (57.2 × 44.5 × 35.6 cm).
- Weight: 64 lb (29 kg).
- Operating environmental temperature: 50–90° F (10–32° C).
- Operating environmental relative humidity: 20% to 95%, noncondensing.
- X-ray source: 60 kV, <0.3 mA.
- X-ray filtration: Tin.
- Detectors: Two solid state.
- Quality control: Automatic with internal phantoms requiring <5 minutes.

- Operation: Handheld console with fluorescent display, unit on wheels with retractable handle, built-in floppy disc drive for data transfer, built-in parallel printer port for Canon BJC color printer or equivalent.
- Options: Laptop configuration.

DexaCare™ DTX-200 (Figs. 4-14 and 4-15)

- Manufacturer: Osteometer MediTech, Hawthorne, CA.
- Technology: Dual-energy X-ray absorptiometry.
- Skeletal application: Forearm.
- Scan time: 4.5 minutes.
- Results
  —BMD (g/cm²).
  —BMC (g).
- Area (cm²).
  —% Young adult and % age-matched comparisons.
  —T-score and z-score.
- Precision: <1%.
- Radiation dose: 0.1 µSv/scan.
- Dimensions: 32 × 24 × 12 in. (80 × 62 × 30 cm).
- Weight: 114 lb (52 kg).
- Environmental operating temperature: 58–86° F (15–30° C).
- X-ray source: 55 kV, 300 µA.
- X-ray filtration: Tin, K-edge filtration.
- Detectors: Solid state.
- Imaging resolution: 0.4 × 0.4 mm.
- Scatter radiation: <0.25 µSv/hour at 1 m.
- Quality control: Automated with forearm phantom supplied by manufacturer.
- Operation: IBM-compatible computer, HP DeskJet 600C or equivalent printer, VGA monitor, unit on wheels for easy mobility.

pDEXA® (Fig. 4-16)

- Norland Medical Systems, Ft. Atkinson, WI.
- Technology: Dual-energy X-ray absorptiometry.
- Skeletal application: Forearm.
- Scan time: <5 minutes.
- Results
  —BMD (g/cm²).
  —BMC (g).
  —Area (cm²).
  —% Young-reference and % age-matched comparisons.

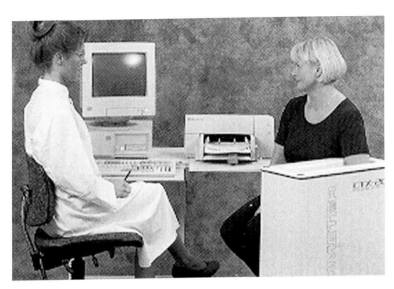

Fig. 4-14. Osteometer DexaCare DTX-200. This is a peripheral dual-energy X-ray absorptiometer used to measure bone density in the forearm. (Photograph courtesy of Osteometer MediTech, Hawthorne, CA.)

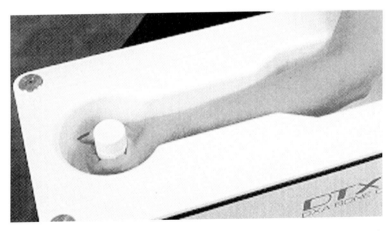

Fig. 4-15. Osteometer DexaCare DTX-200. The forearm is placed into the well in the top of the machine. (Photograph courtesy of Osteometer MediTech, Hawthorne, CA.)

—T-score and z-score.
- Precision: <2.0%.
- Radiation dose: <1.5 mrem at high speed.
- Dimensions: 20.5 × 17 × 16.7 in. (52 × 43 × 42.5 cm).
- Weight: 59.4 lb (27 kg).

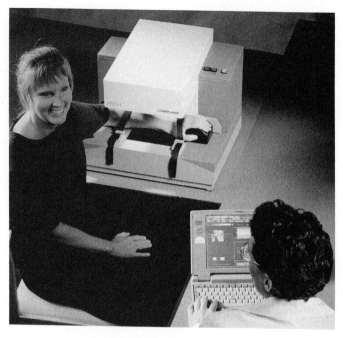

Fig. 4-16. Norland pDEXA. This is a peripheral dual-energy X-ray absorptiometer used to measure bone density in the forearm. (Photograph courtesy of Norland Medical Systems, Ft. Atkinson, WI.)

- Environmental operating temperature: 60–82° F (15–28° C).
- Environmental operating relative humidity: up to 80%, noncondensing.
- X-ray source: 60 kV, <0.3 mA.
- X-ray filtration: Tin.
- Detectors: Two solid state.
- Quality control: Automatic with manufacturer-supplied calibration standard and QC phantom.
- Operation: IBM-compatible laptop computer with Windows operating system, HP DeskJet printer and mouse.
- Options: IBM-compatible desktop computer with Windows operating system, 15-in. SVGA monitor, 15-in. flat panel display, 17-in. SVGA monitor, HP DeskJet.

PIXI® (Peripheral Instantaneous X-ray Imager) (Fig. 4-17)

- Manufacturer: GE Lunar, Madison, WI.
- Technology: Dual-energy X-ray absorptiometry.

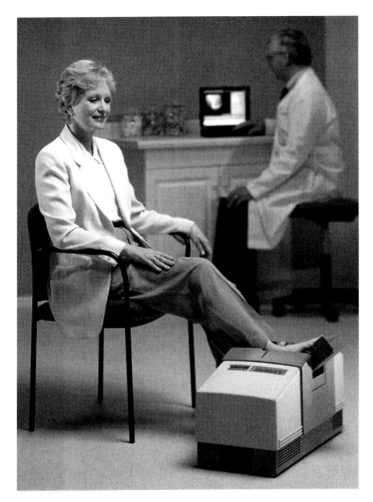

Fig. 4-17. GE Lunar PIXI. This is a peripheral dual-energy X-ray absorptiometer shown here in the configuration used to measure bone density in the calcaneus. The device can be reconfigured and used to measure bone density in the forearm. (Photograph courtesy of GE Lunar, Madison, WI.)

- Skeletal applications: Calcaneus, forearm.
- Scan time: 5 seconds.
- Results
  —BMD (g/cm^2).
  —% Young-adult and % age-matched comparisons.
  —T-score and z-score.
- Precision: <1.5%.

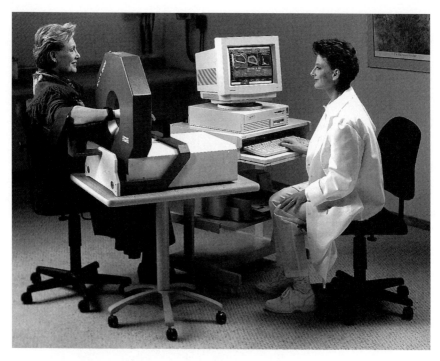

Fig. 4-18. Norland XCT 2000. This is a peripheral quantitative computed tomography device used to measure bone density in the forearm. (Photograph courtesy of Norland Medical Systems, Ft. Atkinson, WI.)

- Radiation dose: 0.032 μSv.
- Dimensions: 12 × 25 × 13 in. (30 × 63 × 33 cm).
- Weight: 66 lb (<30 kg).
- Environmental operating temperature: 64–81° F (18–27° C).
- X-ray source: Cone-beam geometry, 250-μA current.
- Image resolution: 0.2 × 0.2 mm.
- Quality control: Aluminum os calcis and forearm phantoms supplied by the manufacturer.
- Operation: Laptop computer, printer.
- Options: Portable color printer, reusable hard shipping case, soft-sided portability case and cart.

XCT 2000™ (Fig. 4-18)

- Manufacturer: Norland Medical Systems, Ft. Atkinson, WI.
- Technology: Computerized tomography.
- Skeletal application: Forearm.

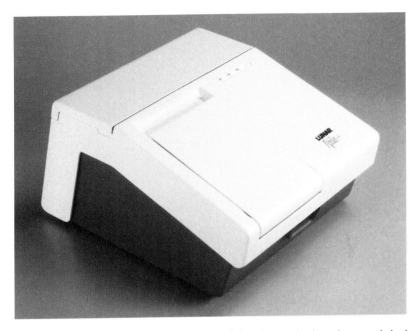

Fig. 4-19. GE Lunar Achilles+. This is a peripheral quantitative ultrasound device used to measure the calcaneus, shown here in the closed position. (Photograph courtesy of GE Lunar, Madison, WI.)

- Scan time: 80 seconds.
- Results: BMD (mg/cm^3) for total bone and trabecular and cortical compartments.
- Precision: ±3 mg/cm^3 for trabecular bone, ±9 mg/cm^3 for cortical bone.
- Radiation dose: 0.03 mSv/scan.
- Dimensions: 21.7 × 36.6 × 24.4 in. (55 × 93 × 62 cm).
- Weight: <100 lb (<45 kg).
- X-ray source: 45 to 49 kV, <0.3 mA.
- Detectors: Six semiconductor detectors with amplifiers.
- Operation: Pentium computer, monitor, and color printer.
- Options: Magneto-opticals for data backup.

ULTRASOUND BONE DENSITOMETERS

Achilles+™ (Figs. 4-19 and 4-20)

- Manufacturer: GE Lunar, Madison, WI.
- Technology

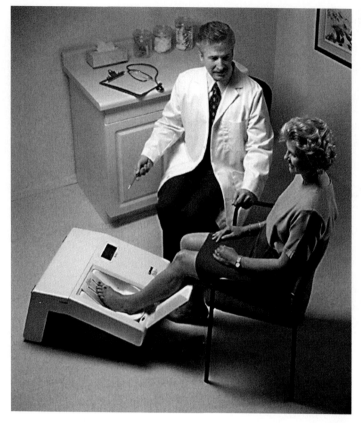

Fig. 4-20. GE Lunar Achilles+ shown in use. (Photograph courtesy of GE Lunar, Madison, WI.)

—Ultrasound.
—Transmitted through bone.
—Wet.
• Skeletal application: Calcaneus.
• Scan time: 1 minute.
• Results
—SOS (m/second).
—BUA (db/MHz).
—Stiffness Index.
—% Young adult and % age-matched comparisons.
—T-score and z-score.
• Precision: 2.0% for Stiffness™ Index.
• Dimensions: 20 × 13 × 24 in. (51 × 33 × 61 cm).

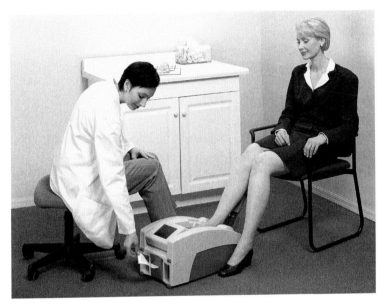

Fig. 4-21. GE Lunar Achilles Express. This is a peripheral quantitative ultrasound device used to measure the calcaneus. (Photograph courtesy of GE Lunar, Madison, WI.)

- Weight: 44 lb (20 kg).
- Operating environmental temperature: 59–95° F (15–35° C).
- Operating environmental relative humidity: 20% to 80%.
- Operation: Self-contained LCD touch screen, thermal printer, 50-measurement memory, built-in carrying handle.
- Accessories provided
  —Water-soluble ultrasonic gel.
  —Premeasured surfactant.
- Options: Laptop computer, external printer.

Achilles Express™ (Fig. 4-21)

- Manufacturer: GE Lunar, Madison, WI.
- Technology
  —Ultrasound.
  —Transmitted through bone.
  —Dry.
- Skeletal applications: Calcaneus.
- Scan time: 1 minute.

- Results
  —Stiffness Index.
  —% Young adult and % age-matched comparisons.
  —T-score and z-score.
- Precision: 2.0%.
- Dimensions: 10 × 12 × 24 in. (25 × 31 × 61 cm).
- Weight: 22 lb (10 kg).
- Operating environmental temperature: 59–95° F (15–35° C).
- Operating environmental relative humidity: 20% to 80%.
- Operation: Self-contained LCD touch screen that swivels, thermal printer, 100-measurement memory, built-in carrying handle.
- Accessories: Water-soluble ultrasonic gel.

McCue C.U.B.A.Clinical™ (Contact Ultrasound Bone Analyzer) (Fig. 4-22)

- Manufacturer: Norland Medical Systems, Ft. Atkinson, WI.
- Technology
  —Ultrasound.
  —Transmitted through bone.
  —Dry.
- Skeletal application: Calcaneus.
- Scan time: 1 minute.
- Results
  —BUA (db/MHz).
  —% Young-reference and % age-matched comparisons.
  —T-score and z-score.
- Precision: 1.3% for BUA.
- Dimensions: 17.8 × 13.9 × 10.2 in. (45.2 × 35.3 × 25.9 cm).
- Weight: 22 lb (10 kg).
- Environmental storage temperature: 23°–122° F (−5° to 50° C).
- Environmental storage humidity: 10% to 95%.
- Quality control: Internal phantom and external quality assurance phantom.
- Operation: IBM-compatible computer with a minimum 10 MB of free hard drive space, 486DX2 microprocessor at 66 MHz, 1.44-MB floppy disc drive, serial port, Windows 3.1 or higher (Windows NT not supported), and Microsoft Windows–supported printer (all computer equipment supplied by end user).
- Accessories provided
  —Padded carrying bag for C.U.B.A.
  —Padded carrying bag for QA phantom, QA phantom.

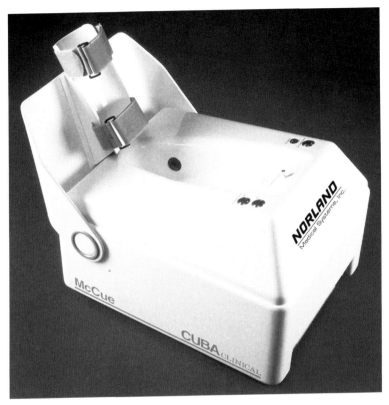

Fig. 4-22. Norland McCue C.U.B.A. Clinical. This is a peripheral quantitative ultrasound device used to measure the calcaneus. (Photograph courtesy of Norland Medical Systems, Ft. Atkinson, WI.)

—Bottle of ultrasound gel.

—Two anatomic foot inserts.

—C.U.B.A. plus+ software.

—Serial cable.

—Power cable.

—User's manual.

Omnisense™ 7000S Ultrasound Bone Sonometer (Figs. 4-23 and 4-24)

- Manufacturer: Sunlight Medical, Rehovot, Israel
- Technology
    —Ultrasound.
    —Axially transmitted along bone.
    —Dry.

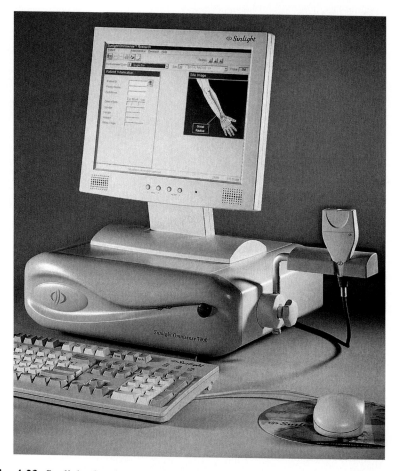

Fig. 4-23. Sunlight Omnisense 7000S. This is a peripheral quantitative ultrasound device used to measure the radius. (Photograph courtesy of Sunlight Medical, Rehovot, Israel.)

- Skeletal applications: Forearm (other regions pending Food and Drug Administration approval).
- Scan time: Approximately 1 minute.
- Results
  —SOS (m/sec).
  —T-score and *z*-score.
- Precision: 0.4%–0.8% as the RMS CV, depending on the site.
- Main unit dimensions: 15.4 × 5.1 × 13 in. (39 × 13 × 33 cm).
- Main unit weight: 15 lb (7 kg).
- Operating environmental temperature: 50–95° F (10–35° C).

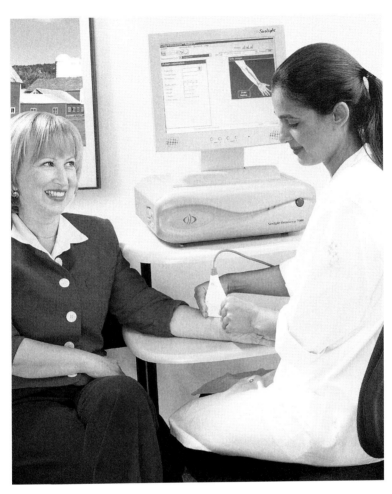

Fig. 4-24. Sunlight Omnisense 7000S shown in use. (Photograph courtesy of Sunlight Medical Ltd., Rehovot, Israel.)

- Operating environmental relative humidity: 30% to 75%, noncondensing.
- Quality control: Calibration free; daily system verification with phantom required.
- Operation: IBM-compatible computer with Windows 95 interface, 14-in. CRT monitor, mouse or trackball, printer.
- Accessories provided
  —System quality verification phantom.
  —Aquasonic® Clear® Ultrasound Gel.
- Options: Flat panel display.

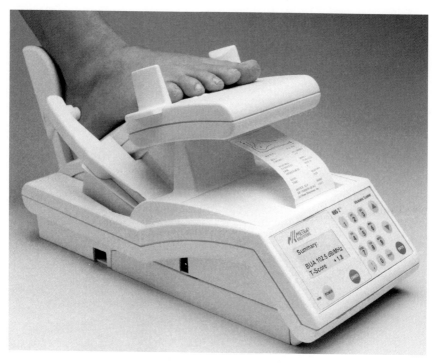

Fig. 4-25. Quidel QUS-2. This is a peripheral quantitative ultrasound device used to measure the calcaneus. (Photograph courtesy of Quidel, Mountain View, CA.)

QUS™-2 (Fig. 4-25)

- Manufacturer: Quidel, Mountain View, CA.
- Technology
  —Ultrasound.
  —Transmitted through bone.
  —Dry.
- Skeletal applications: Calcaneus.
- Scan time: Less than 2 minutes.
- Results
  —BUA (dB/MHz).
  —T-score.
- Precision: 2.6%.
- Dimensions: 7.5 × 16.0 × 9.0 in. (19.1 × 40.6 × 22.9 cm).
- Weight: 7 lb (3.2 kg).
- Environmental operating temperature: 59–95° F (15–35° C).

- Environmental operating relative humidity: 30 to 75%, noncondensing.
- Quality control: Automated with supplied test object.
- Operation: Self-contained unit with messages displayed on LCD screen. The keyboard on the unit allows data entry. Results are printed by an on-board printer. Foot size accommodated ranges from women's shoe size 5 to men's shoe size 12. On-board storage capacity is approximately 8000 scan summary files. An RS232 interface is used to download scan data to a computer.
- Accessories provided
  —QUS-2 power supply.
  —Rechargeable battery.
  —AC cable.
  —Operator's manual.
  —Printer paper.
  —Aqueous gel.
  —Alcohol prep pads.
  —Test object.
- Options: Carrying case.

Sahara Clinical Bone Sonometer® (Figs. 4-26 and 4-27)

- Manufacturer: Hologic, Bedford, MA.
- Technology
  —Ultrasound.
  —Transmitted through bone.
  —Dry.
- Skeletal application: Calcaneus.
- Scan time: <10 seconds.
- Results
  —Estimated BMD (g/cm^2).
  —Quantitative Ultrasound Index (QUI) obtained from BUA and SOS.
  —T-score and z-score.
- Precision
  —BMD: 3% or 0.014 g/cm^2.
  —QUI: 2.6% or 2.2.
- Dimensions: 17 × 14 × 12 in. (43 × 36 × 30 cm).
- Weight: 22 lb (10 kg).
- Environmental operating temperature: 60–100° F (15–37.7° C).
- Environmental operating relative humidity: 20% to 80%, noncondensing.

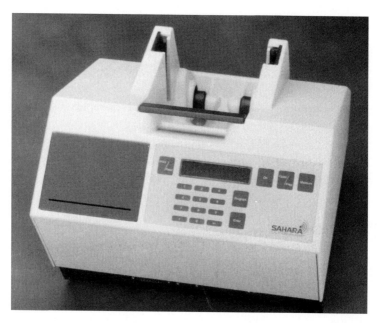

Fig. 4-26. Hologic Sahara Clinical Bone Sonometer. This is a peripheral quantitative ultrasound device used to measure the calcaneus. (Photograph courtesy of Hologic, Bedford, MA.)

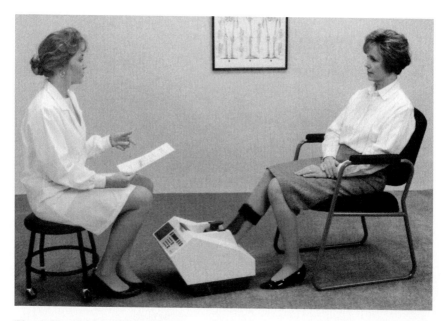

Fig. 4-27. Hologic Sahara Clinical Bone Sonometer shown in use. (Photograph courtesy of Hologic, Bedford, MA.)

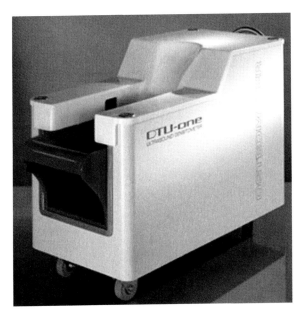

Fig. 4-28. Osteometer Ultrasure DTU-one. This is a peripheral quantitative ultrasound device used to measure the calcaneus. (Photograph courtesy of Osteometer MediTech, Hawthorne, CA.)

- Quality control: Daily, with supplied QC phantom.
- Operation: Embedded microprocessor, data and command input from touch pad on unit, built-in strip printer.
- Accessories provided
  —QC phantom.
  —Sahara coupling gel.
  —Alcohol wipes.
  —Patient report forms.
  —Operator training video.
- Options
  —Carrying case.
  —Spare battery.

UltraSure™ DTU-one (Figs. 4-28 and 4-29)

- Osteometer MediTech, Hawthorne, CA.
- Technology
  —Imaging ultrasound.
  —Transmitted through bone.
  —Wet.

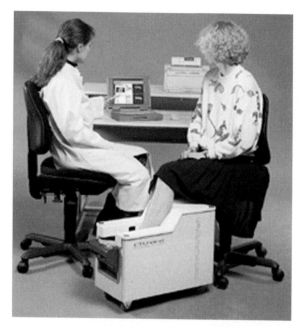

Fig. 4-29. Osteometer Ultrasure DTU-one shown in use. (Photograph courtesy of Osteometer MediTech, Hawthorne, CA.)

- Skeletal application: Calcaneus.
- Scan time: 3 minutes.
- Results
  —SOS (m/second).
  —BUA (dB/MHz).
  —% Young adult and % age-matched comparisons.
  —T-score and z-score.
- Precision
  —SOS: 0.2%.
  —BUA: 1.6%.
- Dimensions: 21 × 11 × 17 in. (53 × 28 × 44 cm).
- Weight: 64 lb (29 kg).
- Environmental operating temperature: 59–86° F (15–30° C).
- Image resolution: 0.6 mm.
- Quality control: Automated with supplied phantom.
- Operation: IBM-compatible Pentium computer with Windows NT operating system, 15-in. SVGA monitor, printer.
- Accessories provided: Phantom

5 Computer Basics

A basic knowledge of computer components, terminology, and functions is not just desirable for a technologist but absolutely necessary in the practice of densitometry today. Appendix XI is a glossary of computer terms that should be part of the vocabulary of the densitometry technologist. In the twenty-first century, dual X-ray absorptiometry, single X-ray absorptiometry, and ultrasound devices are computer driven. Even techniques such as some forms of radiographic absorptiometry and radiogrammetry that require plain skeletal radiographs utilize computer systems with special software to analyze the films. Some peripheral X-ray and ultrasound devices are self-contained; that is, the computer and bone densitometer are blended into one machine. Many of these devices can be configured to operate with a separate computer if the technologist so desires. The use of a separate computer may be desirable when there is a need to store data on many patients for an indefinite period of time. The computers that control the operation of X-ray densitometers are often considered by the Food and Drug Administration (FDA) to be the X-ray controllers. As a consequence, the computer systems used to operate X-ray bone densitometers are sold as part of a package with the densitometer itself. In fact, the use of a nondensitometry manufacturer-supplied computer to operate an X-ray densitometry system may be a violation of FDA regulations. With that said, there is generally nothing special about the computers used to operate densitometers that distinguishes them from a computer that might be found in someone's home.

TYPES OF COMPUTERS

Desktops, Towers, Minitowers, and Laptops

Personal computers are often called *desktops* or *towers,* depending on the size and shape of the computer housing. A desktop computer, as the term implies, is a computer that can be placed comfortably on top of a desk. The term also implies, however, that the computer housing is deeper and wider than it is tall. A tower is a computer that is much taller than it is wide, as shown in Fig. 5-1. A minitower is not quite as tall, but it will still be more tall than wide. Towers and minitowers are usually placed on the floor, but some minitowers are placed on top of a desk. One style of computer housing is not necessarily better than the other. A laptop computer is a portable computer that opens like a notebook to reveal the monitor screen and keyboard. Most laptops weigh 7 lb or less. As laptop technology has improved, the monitor screens on laptops have approached the size of the small screens on monitors used with desktop and tower personal computers. The keyboard on a laptop is necessarily smaller than the full-size keyboards that accompany desktop or tower computers. For the data entry required in performing densitometry, this smaller keyboard generally presents no problems. When typing large amounts of text, however, the full-size keyboard is unquestionably easier to use. Many peripheral densitometers can be purchased with either desktop or tower comput-

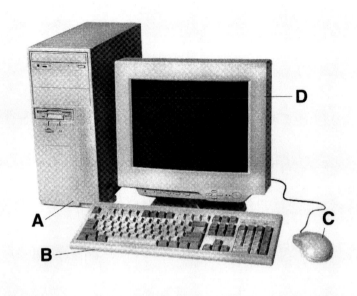

Fig. 5-1. Basic computer system. This is a tower computer (**A**) with a flat panel display monitor (**D**), keyboard (**B**), and mouse (**C**). (Photograph © Hemera Technologies.)

ers or laptops. If portability in the peripheral densitometer is important, a laptop computer instead of a desktop or tower is preferable.

PCs and Macs

In addition to being characterized based on the size and shape of the computer housing, personal computers are also characterized by their operating system. In today's personal computer world, the computers are generally either PCs or Macs. Although *PC* is actually the abbreviation for personal computer, it has become synonymous with an IBM-compatible computer in which the operating system of the computer is either the character-based PC-DOS or MS-DOS. Mac is short for the Macintosh operating system found in computers manufactured by Apple. The Macintosh operating system employs a graphic user interface (GUI) that distinguishes it from the character-based PC-DOS or MS-DOS. Although most PCs now employ the GUI known as Windows, distinct differences exist between the Macintosh and Windows operating systems. Peripheral devices, software utilities, and applications may run on a computer utilizing one type of operating system but not the other. Diskettes must be formatted for one type of system or the other. The computers utilized in densitometry are generally IBM-compatible computers or PCs that utilize DOS or Windows.

MAJOR COMPONENTS OF A COMPUTER SYSTEM

A basic computer system is shown in Fig. 5-1. It is customary to refer to all the various devices as a whole as the computer, but the term *computer* really refers only to device A in Fig. 5-1. The keyboard is device B and the mouse is device C. The keyboard and mouse are both input devices because they are used to "input" information into the computer. Device D in Fig. 5-1 is the monitor. The monitor, keyboard, and mouse are called *peripherals.* Any device that is attached to the computer by a cable or communicates with a computer using radio waves or infrared waves can legitimately be called a peripheral device, including a bone densitometer. All the physical components of a computer system are collectively called *hardware.* This is in contrast to *software,* which refers to the computer programs such as operating systems, utilities, and applications.

Important Components Inside the Computer Housing

MOTHERBOARD, RANDOM ACCESS MEMORY, AND SLOTS

The motherboard found inside the computer housing is illustrated in Fig. 5-2. The motherboard is the main circuit board in the computer. On the motherboard is the microprocessor or central processing unit (CPU) and all the microcircuitry that carries information from the microprocessor to the other components. The hard drive and internal disk drives are also found here. The random access memory (RAM) is located on the motherboard as well. Depending on the particular type of computer, the RAM comprises small boards called SIMMS, DIMMS, or SDRAM. There may be more than one of these, grouped together, depending on the amount of memory found in the computer. There are also slots, called ISA or PCI slots, as shown in Fig. 5-2. Into these slots cards can be inserted to attach different types of peripheral devices to the computer; Fig. 5-3 shows an ISA card. An internal modem card may be found inserted in a slot. Audio cards and video cards may also be present in various card slots. A number of cables will be found on the motherboard, through which the various drives communicate with the CPU.

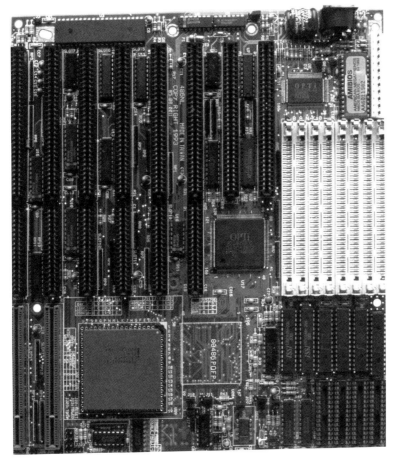

Fig. 5-2. Computer motherboard. (Photograph © 2000 IMS Communications: <www.picture-gallery.com>.)

THE CPU

The CPU, as previously noted, is found on the motherboard inside the computer housing. It is the brain of the computer. In one analogy, the CPU is like the conductor of a symphony orchestra. The conductor directs the interpretation of the music (the software programs) by the members of the orchestra (all the other components and attached peripheral devices). Without the conductor, there would be chaos in the orchestra; without the CPU, the computer can do nothing. CPUs are also often called chips. Major manufacturers include Intel, AMD, and Cyrix. Each manufacturer has different kinds of chips with their own trade names such as Intel's

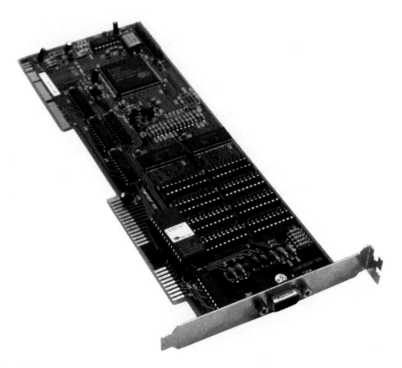

Fig. 5-3. ISA card. (Photograph © 2000 IMS Communications: <www.picture-gallery.com>.)

well-known Celeron and Pentium III chips. CPUs are also characterized by their clock speed, generally measured in megahertz (MHz), although the newest CPUs have speeds measured in gigahertz (GHz). The clock speed reflects the electrical cycles per second sent to the CPU, which essentially controls the rate at which the CPU processes instructions. Today, CPUs found in personal computers commonly have speeds of 500 MHz or higher.

THE HARD DRIVE

The hard drive is the primary data storage medium inside the computer. Because it is inside the computer, it is considered a *fixed* or *internal* storage medium. Today's hard drives can hold an incredible amount of information. Some of the very first personal computers and laptops had hard drives of 20 to 40 MB. Fifteen years ago, this size of hard drive was considered large. A small hard drive today is a 3-GB drive, which can hold 75 times more data than a 40-MB drive. Personal computers commonly have hard drives of 30 GB or more.

Unlike other disk drives and the magnetic or optical storage media that they use, the term *hard drive* refers to both the drive that reads and writes the data and to the magnetic media to which the data are written. The hard drive itself is remarkably similar to an old record player. Inside the hard drive is a round, polished platter that has a magnetic coating. Much like an old 45 or 78 rpm record, the platter has concentric circles on it called tracks that cover the entire surface. The platter is also divided into sectors, which are analogous to slices of pie. When the computer is powered up or *booted,* the platter begins to spin at extremely high speeds. Hanging over the platter is the drive actuator arm, which functions like the needle arm of an old record player. At the end of the drive actuator arm is a device called the read-write head. The head is normally separated from the platter by no more than 2 millionths of an inch and is never supposed to touch the platter. To put this into perspective, a human hair is about 10 millionths of an inch thick. Data are written to the hard drive by an electric current that comes through the write head on the actuator arm and is transmitted to the magnetic coating on the platter. The hard drive is usually assigned the capital letter *C* in computer terminology.

INTERNAL DISK DRIVES

The internal disk drives are drives that are contained within the computer housing but that will open externally to allow the user to insert a diskette or other type of removable storage media into the drive. In this case, the term *disk drive* refers only to the drive and not to the storage media that is used by the drive. Before the advent of zip disks and compact discs (CDs), internal disk drives accommodated diskettes that were either 3½ or 5¼ in. square. Whichever disk drive was uppermost in the computer housing was assigned the lowercase letter *a,* and the other drive was assigned the lowercase letter *b.* The 5¼-in. diskettes are no longer used. Consequently, the 5¼-in. disk drive has largely disappeared from today's computers. The disk drive for 3½-in. diskettes is still traditionally assigned the letter *a,* however, even if it is not the uppermost drive in the computer housing.

There are internal drives for other types of magnetic storage media as well. Zip drives read and write data on zip disks. Tape drives read and write data on magnetic tape and super floppy drives read and write data on super floppies as well as standard floppies. Optical drives employ a laser to read indentations or pits on a CD. The pits reflect varying degrees of light, which are translated into information that the computer can understand. A CD-ROM drive that will read data or play audio from a

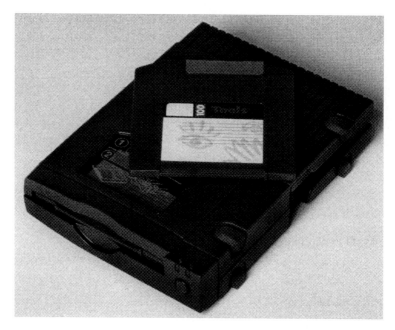

Fig. 5-4. External zip drive and zip disk. (Photograph © Hemera Technologies.)

CD-ROM is a type of optical drive. Some of the newest internal optical drives are CD-R and CD-RW drives, which not only read data and play audio from CD-ROM disks but also read and write data and audio on a new type of CD called either a CD-R or CD-RW. In a CD-R or CD-RW drive, the laser actually heats a dye on the CD, causing less light to be reflected at that location. The effect is the same as the pit created on a CD-ROM. The differences in light reflectivity are translated into digital information when the disk is read.

These magnetic and optical drives are assigned letters of their own, which can be any letter other than *C* or *a*. If these drives are not present inside the computer housing, but instead are attached to the computer by a cable, they are called external disk drives. An external zip drive is shown in Fig. 5-4.

Input Devices

The Keyboard

The basic layout of the alphabetical and numerical keys on the computer keyboard shown in Fig. 5-5 is the same as found on old QWERTY

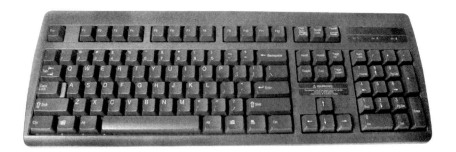

Fig. 5-5. Computer keyboard. (Photograph © Hemera Technologies.)

typewriters. The keys of the QWERTY typewriter account for only 54 of the 104 keys found on standard computer keyboards. The keys on the top row of the keyboard are called *function keys*. They are numbered F1 through F12. These keys have different actions depending on the software program being run. Other special keys found on the bottom row include the control key, abbreviated *Ctrl,* and the alternate key, abbreviated *Alt.* On laptop computer keyboards, a Function key, abbreviated *Fn,* is also found. These keys are depressed in combination with other keys in order to initiate a particular action. Another special key is the escape key, abbreviated *Esc,* found on the top row on the far left. This key, when depressed, generally stops an action or returns the user to the previous viewing screen. In one densitometry manufacturer's software program, however, the Esc key is used to advance the user to the next screen in the program.

There are three other groups of keys, which are normally set apart from the alphabetical and numerical keys on a full-size keyboard. On laptop keyboards, these separate groups may be absent, but their functions are replicated by depressing certain alphabetical keys in combination with the Fn key. The first group is simply a separate set of numerical keys and functions such as found on a calculator. The second group are keys labeled *Page Up, Page Down, Insert, Delete, Home,* and *End.* These keys, again, have different functions depending on the software program being run. Finally, there is a group of keys called *arrow keys.* This is a set of four keys with arrows pointing up, down, right, and left. These keys can be used in a variety of ways, depending on the software program being run but generally initiate some type of directional action.

There are also three special keys found on the bottom row of keyboards for computer systems using the Windows operating system. Two of these keys have the Windows logo on them and the third key has a document logo on it. Once again, these keys have slightly different actions depending on the particular software being run. Two other keys are worth noting, only because they are so commonly confused. The backslash key, or "\" key, and the forward slash key, or "/" key, are often used in computer commands and Web addresses. They mean very different things to a computer and must not be interchanged. In recent years, even more keys have been added to full-size computer keyboards. These keys usually have specific functions to facilitate use of the Internet.

The Mouse

In early computers all computer commands were character based; that is, they were entered by typing characters found on the keyboard. The development of GUIs made it possible for a whole series of commands to be initiated by simply activating a single graphic symbol. This was simpler and faster than typing in a series of characters from the keyboard and also eliminated the need to be familiar with the location of the various keys. One simply needed a device that could be used to point to the graphic symbol on the screen and then activate it. This is exactly what is done with the mouse, labeled *C* in Fig. 5-1. It is used to point at the graphic symbol, and, then, by depressing a button on the mouse either once or twice in succession, the series of commands represented by the symbol is initiated.

A mouse generally has two buttons, designated left and right. The left mouse button is the one most often used to initiate programs as well as other actions. The left mouse button rests under the index finger of a right-handed person, making it easier to use. The right mouse button tends to be reserved for specialized actions that differ depending on the program being run. It is usually possible to change which button is used for most functions if the user is left-handed and wishes to do so. Newer mice also have a wheel, which can be used in word processor and spreadsheet programs to move or scroll through documents quickly. This type of mouse is often called a *wheel mouse*.

The Trackball

Trackballs perform exactly the same function as mice. The arrow on the screen is moved by rolling the trackball within its holder rather than by moving a mouse across a surface. The advantage of a trackball is that the holder remains stationery no matter how much the trackball is moved, so the space required for a trackball is less than required for a mouse, which must be rolled around on a desktop surface. If desktop space is limited, a trackball may be preferable to a mouse. There are buttons on the trackball holder that mimic the left and right buttons on a mouse, and some new trackballs also have a wheel.

The keyboard and mouse or trackball are the main input devices for every computer. They generally attach to the computer by a cable, each having a specialized connection or port on the back of the computer. There are keyboards and mice, however, that can use either radio waves or infrared waves to communicate with the computer, eliminating the need for a cable connection.

Output Devices

MONITORS

Monitors are peripheral output devices. While much more emphasis is generally placed on the internal components of the computer system than the monitor, it is the monitor on which the work is displayed. A poor-quality monitor can make working on an otherwise superb computer quite frustrating. Monitor sizes are described like televisions. The dimension that is given is the diagonal dimension of the viewing area given in inches. Some manufacturers provide two measurements: the diagonal dimension of the screen and the diagonal dimension of the casing surrounding the screen. For example, a monitor may be described as a 19-in. monitor with a 17-in. viewable image size. This means that the diagonal dimension of the casing surrounding the screen is 19 in. while the actual viewing screen has a diagonal dimension of 17 in. Equally important is the resolution of the display, which is usually described as the number of dots per square inch (dpi). A monitor with a resolution of 1024 × 768 is a monitor with a horizontal dpi of 1024 and a vertical dpi of 768. With higher resolutions, more information can be seen on any one screen. Dot pitch and vertical scan refresh rate are two other important characteristics of a monitor. The dot pitch in millimeters is the distance between two pixels of the same color on the monitor screen. The smaller the distance, the sharper the image. An example of a dot pitch measurement is 0.25 mm. The vertical scan refresh rate is the number of times per second that the entire screen is refreshed or renewed. This is measured in hertz (Hz). A higher refresh rate results in less screen dimming and flickering. An example of a vertical scan refresh rate is a measurement of 48 to 120 Hz.

Most monitors employ cathode ray tube (CRT) technology in which magnetic fields control the patterns created by electrons on the viewing screen. New monitors employ liquid crystal display (LCD) technology. LCD technology was employed in the screens in laptops long before it was incorporated into full-size monitors for personal computers. With LCD technology, the screen can be flat rather than curved, giving rise to the term *flat panel display* monitor. LCD screens employ active or passive matrix technology. Active-matrix technology is also called *thin film transistor* (TFT) technology. In TFT, transistors control each pixel on the screen, making these screens much brighter and more colorful than passive-matrix technology. TFT flat panel displays also tend to be the most expensive. Flat panel LCD monitors with 15-in. screens are becoming more common, whereas larger flat panel monitors still tend to be rather expensive. Flat panel LCD monitors are smaller overall than comparable CRT monitors with the same size screen. In addition, they weigh much less and require less space on the desktop.

Monitors should be turned off when not in use, even if the computer is left on. In the past, it was imperative that the monitor be turned off to avoid an image being burned into the screen. This is no longer the case, but there is no justification for wasting the electricity. The screens should be kept clean but should only be cleaned with soft, lint-free, antistatic cloths. Depending on the location of the monitor and the lighting in the room, a glare screen may help improve viewing.

PRINTERS

Printers are peripheral output devices that usually communicate with the computer through the parallel port. Some of the earliest printers were dot-matrix and daisy wheel printers, neither commonly used today. Dot-matrix printers printed characters as a series of dots. Daisy wheel printers used a wheel that rotated to print characters. Most printers in use today are inkjet or laser printers. Inkjet printers actually embed ink into the paper. These printers use ink cartridges of various colors that must be replaced as the ink is consumed. Print and graphics quality with inkjet printers is excellent, but the use of poor-quality paper can result in the ink bleeding into the paper, reducing the clarity of the text or image. Laser printers tend to be more expensive than inkjet printers. They use a laser beam to generate an image that is then transferred to paper by using an electrostatic charge to put toner or ink on the paper.

Several factors should be considered when purchasing a printer. Overall cost is always a consideration, but beyond that the resolution and speed of the printer should be considered as well. Printer resolution is given in dots per inch. This refers to how many dots can be placed in one square inch. For text, a resolution of 600 dpi is desirable. For graphics, a higher minimum resolution of 1200×600 dpi is preferred. Color pages take longer to print than black-and-white pages, and graphics generally take longer to print than text. Print speeds can vary by model, so the primary use of the printer should be considered before purchasing a printer. Most densitometry reports contain both text and graphics and some color as well as black text. In the past, the cable that attached the printer to the computer was sold with the printer. This is no longer the case, so printer cables must be purchased separately. The printer specifications should be checked to determine what type of cable is recommended by the printer manufacturer. If the printer is purchased as part of the densitometry system, the printer cable should be supplied as part of the purchase.

COMPUTER PORTS

The various ports to which the cables from peripheral devices and the computer power cable attach are found on the back of the computer housing. Each type of port has a reasonably consistent appearance from computer to computer. Different devices utilize the same type of port from computer to computer as well. Ports and the cable plugs that attach to them are typically described as male or female, depending on whether they have pins or pin receptacles. Care must always be taken when attaching cable plugs to ports to ensure that the pins are correctly oriented to the pin receptacles to avoid bending the pins and permanently damaging either the port or cable plug.

Keyboard and Mouse Ports

As noted earlier, there are usually specific, dedicated ports for the keyboard and mouse cable. These ports are very similar in appearance and are often next to each other. Care must be taken to ensure that the correct cable is plugged into the correct port. Figure 5-6 shows a typical keyboard or mouse port, which is a female port. The mouse port is often called a PS/2 port. This style of port was originally introduced by IBM in its PS/2 line of computers and came to be known as a PS/2 port. It has since become the standard style mouse port on all manufacturers' computers.

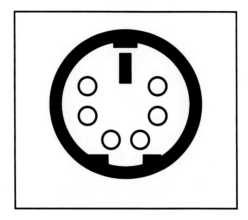

Fig. 5-6. Keyboard or mouse port. This is the standard PS/2 port. The keyboard and mouse each have its own port. Although identical in appearance, they are not interchangeable.

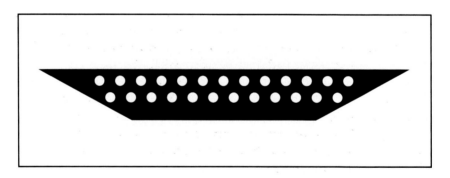

Fig. 5-7. Parallel port. Often used to connect printers to the computer, this is a 25-pin receptacle, female port.

Parallel Ports

The parallel port, as illustrated in Fig. 5-7, is also a female port. It is called a parallel port because it is used by cables having parallel wires. Parallel ports generally have two rows of pin receptacles for a total of 25 receptacles. Parallel ports are commonly used to connect printers to the computer. Computers may have more than one parallel port, in which case the ports are designated as LPT1, LPT2, and so on.

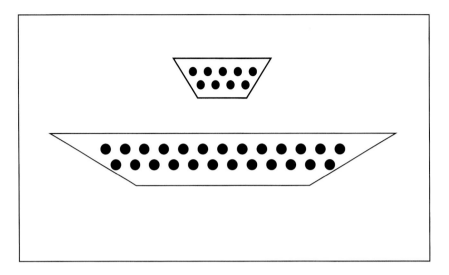

Fig. 5-8. 9-pin and 25-pin serial port. Densitometers often communicate with the computer through the serial port. Adapters can be purchased to change the 9-pin port to a 25-pin port, or the 25-pin port to a 9-pin port.

Serial Ports

Serial ports are male ports, with two rows of pins totaling either 9 or 25, as shown in Fig. 5-8. Computers typically have more than one serial port, which are designated COM1, COM2, and so on, as necessary. A variety of different devices may utilize a serial port. Bone densitometers generally communicate with the computer through a serial port. If a computer has a 9-pin serial port and a device requires a 25-pin serial port, an adapter can be purchased that will convert the 9-pin port to a 25-pin port. The reverse is also true if a computer has a 25-pin port and a 9-pin port is required.

Universal Serial Bus Ports

Universal serial bus (USB) ports are relatively new. Their appearance is quite different from that of parallel and serial ports, as shown in Fig. 5-9. USB ports are designed to enable the computer to communicate with devices using USB architecture. USB is a different type of communication language that was intended to simplify the installation of various devices. It was thought that the USB would replace the other bus architectures or

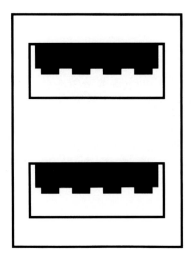

Fig. 5-9. USB port. Many new peripheral devices utilize the USB port.

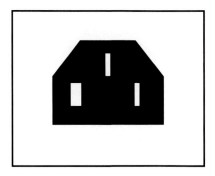

Fig. 5-10. Computer power cord port.

languages used by peripheral devices that required special cards to be inserted into slots in the computer before the device could be attached to the computer. This certainly has not happened yet.

Power, Monitor, Modem, and Network Ports

Other, perhaps more recognizable ports are shown in Fig. 5-10 and 5-11. The power cord outlet port looks very much like a wall socket for any electrical cord. The modem port looks like a typical wall telephone

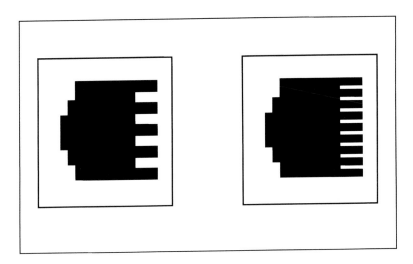

Fig. 5-11. Modem and network communication ports. These two ports are similar in appearance but the network port has twice as many pin receptacles as the modem port. Care must be taken not to confuse the two ports.

jack. One end of the telephone cable is inserted into this port and the other end into the wall jack. The network interface port is very similar in appearance to the modem port, but there are twice as many pin receptacles than found in the modem port. The network interface port is used to connect the computer to a network, rather than a telephone line. Care must be taken not to confuse the two communication ports because damage could result to both the port and telephone line. The monitor also has its own port, shown in Fig. 5-12.

TYPES OF STORAGE MEDIA

Storage media is the media onto which data are written. There are three basic types: magnetic, tape, and optical. Although optical storage media is becoming increasingly popular, magnetic storage media is still the mainstay for data storage.

Magnetic Media

The hard drive is a type of magnetic storage media. The most common magnetic media is the floppy diskette, often simply called a floppy, shown

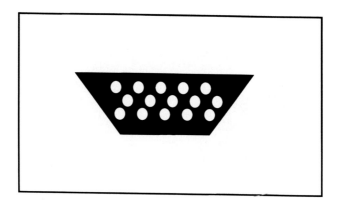

Fig. 5-12. VGA port. The monitor cable attaches here. This is a female port with three rows of pin receptacles.

in Fig. 5-13. In spite of the name, a standard floppy diskette is actually quite hard. It measures about 3½ × 3¹¹/₁₆ × ⅛ in. This size diskette is known as a 3½-in. floppy. The average 3½-in. floppy holds 1.44 MB of data but in the vernacular is called a 1-MB floppy. In the past, a similar physically sized floppy diskette was available that would only hold 750 KB of data. These were called double-sided, double-density diskettes or DS, DD for short. The 1-MB diskettes were called double-sided, high-density diskettes or DS, HD, in order to distinguish them from the otherwise outwardly identical DS, DD disks. Today, most 3½-in. floppies are the 1-MB disks, but the HD designation on the diskette remains, as shown in Fig. 5-13. Floppy diskettes come in all colors, besides basic black. They also are generally preformatted for either IBM-compatible or Macintosh computers. In the past, diskettes were not formatted, requiring the user to do so before data could be written to the diskette. When formatted diskettes became available, they were slightly more expensive than nonformatted diskettes. Today, almost all 3½-in. diskettes are already formatted for either IBM-compatible or Macintosh computers. The type of computer for which they have been formatted is noted on the box. Because most densitometer computers utilize IBM-compatible computers or PCs, they also utilize IBM-formatted diskettes.

On the floppy diskette there are two physical items to inspect. There is a metal door on each floppy that slides back to give the disk drive access to the magnetic media inside the diskette. This door should slide easily. If the door is bent or does not slide easily, it should not be used because it may damage the disk drive. The small tab on the back of the

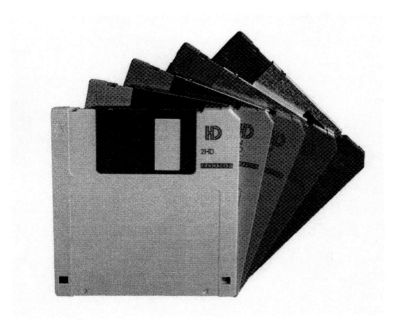

Fig. 5-13. Standard 1.44-MB, 3½-in. floppy disks. The designation HD can be seen in the upper right-hand corner. The read-write protect tab is seen on the lower left and is accessible from the back of the disk. (Photograph © Hemera Technologies.)

diskette at the bottom, called the *write-protect tab,* should be checked to ensure that it is in the proper position. In the up or write position, data can be written to the diskette. In the down or protect position, data cannot be written or erased from the diskette.

There is also a diskette called a *super floppy.* These are diskettes that are roughly the same size as the 3½-in. standard floppy but that hold 120 MB or more of data. To use super floppies, the computer must have a disk drive that is specifically designed for that type of super floppy. Such drives also are generally able to read standard 3½-in. 1 MB floppy disks. Super floppies are a type of magnetic storage media, although optical technology is used to read and write data to the diskette.

A zip disk is another type of diskette with a far greater storage capacity than a standard floppy, measuring roughly 3⅞ in. square × ¼ in. thick. A zip disk is shown in Fig. 5-4. Zip disks cannot be used in floppy disk drives. A specific zip drive must be available, either installed as an internal drive in the computer or attached to the computer as a peripheral device. Zip disks come in either 100-MB or 250-MB sizes. This means that one zip disk can hold an amount of data equivalent to 100 or 250 1-MB standard floppy diskettes. If the 250-MB zip disks are used, the zip drive must be a 250-MB zip disk drive. This drive also reads 100-MB zip disks. The 100-MB zip disk drive only reads 100-MB zip disks. Zip disk drives cannot read standard or super floppy disks. Like floppy diskettes, zip disks are preformatted for either IBM-compatible computers or Macs.

Super floppies and zip disks enable the storage of a much greater amount of data on one diskette when compared with a standard 1-MB floppy. They are more expensive than the standard 3½-in. floppy diskette, but the increase in price is generally proportional to the number of standard floppies that they replace. The upside is that they allow the user to store a great deal of information in one place. The downside is that they cost more per diskette, require specific disk drives, and, if damaged, result in the loss of a lot of information rather than a little. They are particularly useful for storing graphics files, which are often very large files, easily exceeding the 1-MB storage capacity of the standard floppy. Diskettes of any kind should never be stored near magnets or stereo speakers. They also should be protected from extreme heat and never packed tightly together once used. They should not be left in disk drives when not in use. While this is not necessarily bad for the diskette, it causes the drive door to remain open, unnecessarily exposing the drive to dust and other debris.

Tape Media

Magnetic tape is primarily used for backing up data, rather than routine data storage. Tape cartridges, somewhat larger than the standard audiocassette, come in a variety of storage sizes, ranging from several hundred megabytes to several gigabytes. The tape drive can be either internal or external. Utilizing the tape drive and tape cartridge requires software designed to be used with the specific tape drive, unlike other magnetic storage media drives.

Optical Media

CD-ROMs are compact discs from which data can only be read. Although a CD-ROM can hold an enormous amount of data, the user cannot write data to the CD. CD-Rs and CD-RWs are new types of CDs to which the user can write data. The computer must have a CD-R or CD-RW drive to use this type of media. An enormous amount of data can be stored on a single disk, as much as 650 MB. The CD-writable, or CD-R, disc allows data to be written to it only once. The CD-rewritable,

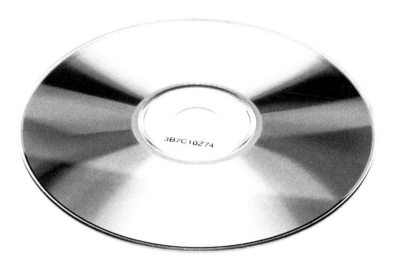

Fig. 5-14. CD-ROM. The appearance of CD-R and CD-RW discs is basically identical. (Photograph © 2000 IMS Communications Ltd: <www.picture-gallery.com>.)

or CD-RW, disc can be erased and rewritten thousands of times. CD-R and CD-RW discs can be read by a regular CD-ROM drive. Similarly, a CD-R drive or a CD-RW drive can read CD-ROMs as well as CD-Rs and CD-RWs. The outward appearance of CD-Rs and CD-RWs is almost indistinguishable from that of the CD-ROM, shown in Fig. 5-14. The back of the CD-R or CD-RW disc, where the data are written, reflects the color of the dye used on the disc.

CDs in general are very durable but they should always be handled by the edges to avoid damaging the read/write surface. Special cloths are available to clean dusty CDs without scratching them. CDs should be stored in plastic cases when not in use. With proper care, the expected life span of a CD-RW disc is 30 years. For a CD-R, the expected life span is 100 years. Either way, the data on them should be preserved for a very long time.

PROTECTING THE DATA

The hard drive inside the computer is the primary location for data storage, but it should never be the only location. It is absolutely imperative that the technologist both backup and archive data from the hard drive. Copies should be made of the backup and archive media. The original and copied backup and archive media should be stored in two different locations. Remember: backup, archive, copy, and separate. Why?

The data should be backed up and copied to protect the data from being lost should some disaster befall the hard drive. The backup and archive media should be copied because they too can eventually be damaged, resulting in an irretrievable loss of data. The copies should be stored in separate locations so that if a physical disaster occurs, such as a fire or flood, the chances of one set surviving are improved.

Hard drives are built to endure a lot of wear and tear. The term *crash* is often used to describe any and every problem that might occur with the hard drive or computer, in general. Originally, however, the term referred to the circumstance in which the read/write head made contact with the hard drive platter, where data were stored. This is similar to dropping the needle arm of a record player onto the record itself. The track on the record where the needle hit would be damaged and the record would skip when it was played. A similar loss of data will occur where the hard drive is touched by the head. Hard drive crashes are fortunately rare in today's computers. Hard drives are sealed to keep out dust, hair, smoke, and other unwanted particles. The platters are coated with a much firmer material than they used to be, making them more resistant to gouging by the heads. It is still possible to jar the hard drive enough to cause the head to damage the platter, but it takes some effort. Nevertheless, it should go without saying that dropping the computer is a very bad idea. Hard drives can eventually fail, however. Failure to back up and copy the data is to court disaster.

Temperature extremes and high humidity are detrimental to hard drives as well as densitometers. The ambient temperature and humidity in the room in which the computer and bone densitometer are housed need to be kept within the ranges specified by the manufacturer. A combination thermometer-hygrometer can generally be purchased at hardware stores for less than $20. Because densitometers also have specific temperature and humidity operating ranges,* such a device is a wise investment to ensure that the computer and densitometer are protected.

Hard drives can also be irreparably damaged by power surges and static discharges. The shutdown sequence required by the operating system should always be followed whenever possible. To this end, surge protectors and uninterruptible power supply (UPS) units are absolute necessities.

---

*See Chapter 4 for the environmental operating temperature and humidity ranges for bone densitometers.

Surge protectors protect the devices plugged into it from electrical spikes or power surges. A surge protector is plugged into a wall outlet and then the computer and its peripheral devices are plugged into the surge protector. The amount of protection offered by a surge protector varies depending on the model. UPS units are a form of backup power for the computer that, in case of a power outage, will continue to provide power to the computer to allow the user to shut down the computer properly and avoid the loss of any data. A UPS unit provides 10–30 minutes of power, depending on the particular model. Some UPS units also provide surge protection for the computer, monitor, and modem or network connections. Remember to keep all forms of magnets away from the computer and magnetic storage media.

COMPUTER MAINTENANCE

Some general computer system maintenance is advisable. The computer and its peripherals should be turned off when not in use. Some years ago it was thought that booting up the computer caused wear and tear on the hard drive, so users would leave the computer on for days at a time, rather than shut down and boot up on a daily basis. This is unnecessary and simply wastes electricity. Scandisk programs (programs that check for errors on the hard drive) should be run often, although how often depends on how much the computer is used. Similarly, disk defragmenter programs (programs that organize or tidy up the file storage) should also be run periodically. If the computer is used daily with frequent installation and uninstallation of programs and downloading of files from the Internet, scandisk and defragmenter programs should be run once a week and at least twice a year, respectively. If this type of activity is infrequent, once a month will suffice for a scandisk program and perhaps once a year for a defragmenter program. Make sure that the computer and every peripheral device has surge protection at all times. If the computer has a modem, utilize a surge protector that also offers protection for telephone lines, because these lines can carry an electrical surge as well as the power cable itself. Surge protectors and UPS units must generally be purchased separately from the computer system but are wise safeguards against equipment damage and data loss, particularly in areas that experience frequent thunderstorms.

There are very few if any user-serviceable components inside the computer housing. Although opening the housing is quite safe when done properly, there is little that the average user can accomplish in the way

of repairs when something goes wrong. Some general preventive maintenance that does require opening the computer housing should be done
once or twice a year. Dust and debris can accumulate inside the housing
and are detrimental to the computer components. Cans of compressed air
or ozone-safe compounds such as tetrafluoroethane can be purchased and
used to blow out the dust and debris safely. It is imperative that the user
be grounded when the computer housing is opened before touching any
part of the interior. This can be accomplished by touching some nonpainted
metal surface. Many computers that accompany bone densitometers have
dire warnings attached that the warranty will be voided if the computer
housing is opened. If this warning is present, call the densitometry manufacturer technical support division and ask permission to open the housing
without voiding the warranty.

Make sure that the openings on the back of the computer housing that
allow air in are not blocked. Today's microprocessors generate heat that
must be dissipated or the computer will crash. This is accomplished by
cooling fans that draw cool air in through the vents and send hot air out.
If the vents are blocked, either by dust and debris or by the computer
being placed too close to a wall, this necessary cooling will not occur.
In the absence of proper cooling either due to blocked vents or fan failure,
the computer itself will crash in only 15 or 20 minutes. The gentle humming
or whirring noise that is usually heard when the computer is in operation
is the sound of the cooling fan. Learn this sound. If this sound is not
normal, it is cause for immediate concern because it may indicate failure
of the fan and imminent disaster for the computer. In this case, back up
the data and obtain professional assistance immediately.

6 Precision in Bone Densitometry

Precision is the attribute of a quantitative measurement technique such as bone densitometry that refers to the ability to reproduce the same numerical result in the setting of no real biological change when the test is repeatedly performed in an identical fashion. Like all quantitative tests in clinical medicine, no bone densitometry technique is perfectly reproducible. This is true even when the bone density test is performed in exact accordance with the manufacturer's recommendations every time. If the technologist does not position the patient and analyze the data in a consistent fashion, the technique becomes even less reproducible.

The precision of bone density testing assumes great importance when the technique is being used to follow changes in bone density over time. Because densitometry is not perfectly reproducible, the results on any given patient are not expected to be identical, even if the bone density in the patient has not actually changed. The only way, then, that a physician can know when a real biological change has occurred is to know when the precision error of the technique has been exceeded. This means that the precision must be quantified by performing a precision study. The precision, which can be given as the standard deviation (SD) with the same units as the measurement, or as the percentage coefficient of variation (%CV), is then used to determine the minimum change in bone density that constitutes a real biological change. This is called the least significant change (LSC). The LSC can then be used to determine the minimum interval between follow-up measurements.

PERFORMING A PRECISION STUDY

The results of three posteroanterior (PA) lumbar spine dual-energy X-ray absorptiometry (DXA) measurements of bone density are shown in Table 6-1. These measurements on the patient Mrs. B were all performed within a few minutes of each other, with only enough time between studies to allow Mrs. B to get off the scan table and be repositioned by the technologist. The same technologist positioned Mrs. B for all three studies and also analyzed all three studies according to the manufacturer's recommendations. For this example, it is reasonable to assume that the technologist performed both tasks perfectly and consistently for all three studies.

Note that the numerical results of the three studies are not identical, even though the tests were conducted perfectly and no biological change could have occurred in Mrs. B in the brief period that elapsed between tests. This reflects the imperfect precision of bone densitometry. A reasonable first step in looking at Mrs. B's measurements in Table 6-1 is to ask, What is the average or mean value of the three measurements? This value is calculated by adding the values from the three individual measurements and dividing the total by 3. The average value for the set of three measurements on Mrs. B was 1.021 g/cm^2. The next question that must be answered is, By how much do each of the three measurements vary from the mean value? This can be found by subtracting each of the three actual measurements from the mean value, as shown in Eqs. 1–3.

$$\text{Study no. 1: } 1.021 \text{ g/cm}^2 - 1.011 \text{ g/cm}^2 = 0.010 \text{ g/cm}^2 \qquad (1)$$
$$\text{Study no. 2: } 1.021 \text{ g/cm}^2 - 1.030 \text{ g/cm}^2 = -0.009 \text{ g/cm}^2 \qquad (2)$$
$$\text{Study no. 3: } 1.021 \text{ g/cm}^2 - 1.022 \text{ g/cm}^2 = -0.001 \text{ g/cm}^2 \qquad (3)$$

It would seem reasonable at this point to ask what the representative variation is from the mean for each of these measurements. An intuitive approach would be to find the average difference by adding the three differences found in Eqs. 1–3 and dividing the sum by 3. This is not

Table 6-1
Results of Precision Study on Mrs. B

PA spine DXA study	Value
Study no. 1	1.011 g/cm²
Study no. 2	1.030 g/cm²
Study no. 3	1.022 g/cm²
Mean	1.021 g/cm²
SD	0.010 g/cm²
%CV	1.0

mathematically possible, however. Note that if the three differences were added, they would total 0, which cannot be divided. Instead, the formula shown in Eq. 4 is used. The three differences are squared, to remove the minus signs. After squaring, they are added and the resulting total is divided by the number of measurements minus 1 (or in this case 2). The square root is then taken. The resulting value is called the standard deviation (SD) for the set of three measurements on Mrs. B. The SD has the units of the measurement (g/cm²), and is the appropriate expression of the representative variability about the mean for the three measurements on Mrs. B. The SD is also the appropriate expression of the precision of the three measurements.

$$\text{SD}_B = \sqrt{\frac{\sum_{i=1}^{n_B} (X_{iB} - \overline{X}_B)^2}{n_B - 1}} \qquad (4)$$

In Eq. 4, n_B is the number of measurements on Mrs. B, X_{iB} is the actual value of the ith measurement on Mrs. B, and $\overline{X}_B$ (pronounced "ex bar") is the mean bone mineral density (BMD) value for Mrs. B. The sum of the squared differences is divided by $n - 1$ rather than n because, in this case, only two of the three measurements actually contribute independently to the calculation of the mean. In other words, if the average value and two of the three measured values that were used to calculate the average were known, the third measured value could always be determined mathematically. The third value is thus not independent. In the example presented, the SD for the set of three measurements on Mrs. B is 0.010 g/cm², as shown in Table 6-1.

Now that the SD and mean value for the three measurements on Mrs. B are known to be 0.010 and 1.021 g/cm², respectively, it can be asked, What proportion or percentage of the mean does the SD represent? This

Table 6-2
Combination of Number of Patients and Scans/Patient
for a Statistically Valid Precision Study

No. of patients	No. of scans/patient
1	31
5	7
10	4
15	3
30	2

is found by dividing the SD by the mean as shown in Eq. 5. This quantity is the coefficient of variation (CV). When multiplied by 100 and expressed as a percentage, it is the percent coefficient of variation (%CV), as shown in Eq. 6. The CV and %CV are alternative expressions of the precision of the measurement. For Mrs. B, the CV was 0.01 and the %CV, 1%.

$$CV = SD/\overline{X} \tag{5}$$
$$\%CV = (SD/\overline{X}) \times 100 \tag{6}$$

Although the SD, CV, or %CV for Mrs. B could be used in determining significant changes in PA lumbar spine bone density over time for Mrs. B, calculating individual precision values for each patient that might be followed over time is not practical. It is necessary to establish representative precision values for each skeletal site used for monitoring at a bone densitometry facility. This can be done by performing a short-term precision study.

Short-Term Precision Studies

A separate precision study should be done for each skeletal site that might be used in following a patient. Table 6-2 gives the specific combinations of the number of patients and number of scans per patient that are recommended for a short-term precision study.

Remember that one of the measurements on an individual will not contribute independently to the calculation of the mean for that individual. The number that does independently contribute is called the degrees of freedom (df) for the study. For statistical validity, it is recommended that a short-term precision study have 30 df (1). If only one person is studied, 31 tests must be performed to obtain 30 df because one test will not contribute independently to the calculation of the mean. If 10 patients are studied, four tests per patient must be done because, again, only three of the four tests per patient will be independent ($10 \times 3 = 30$). Thirty degrees of freedom is chosen to ensure that the upper limit for the 95% confidence interval (CI) of the precision value that is calculated is no more than 34% greater than the calculated precision value. A short-term precision study should be completed in 2 weeks to 1 month. All the scans on any one patient can be completed on the same day if desired.

Using the combination of 10 patients and four scans each for the sake of example, the average value, SD, and CV should be found for each of the 10 sets of four measurements, just as was done for the set of three measurements on Mrs. B. Rather than reporting the arithmetic mean of the 10 SDs or 10 CVs (adding the 10 values and dividing by 10) as the precision value, the root-mean-square SD (RMS-SD) or the root-mean-square CV (RMS-CV) is calculated as shown in Eqs. 7 and 8 (2):

$$SD_{RMS} = \sqrt{\frac{\sum_{i=1}^{m} (SD^2)}{m}} \tag{7}$$

$$CV_{RMS} = \sqrt{\frac{\sum_{i=1}^{m} (CV^2)}{m}} \tag{8}$$

in which m is the number of patients. Using these equations, the 10 SDs or 10 CVs are squared, summed, and then divided by the number of patients, 10. Then the square root is taken, resulting in the RMS-SD or RMS-CV for the group of 10 patients. The RMS-SD or RMS-CV is the preferred expression of the short-term precision at any skeletal site. The RMS-CV can be expressed as a percentage, the RMS-%CV, by multiplying by 100.

Long-Term Precision Studies

A long-term precision study in which patients are followed over the course of at least a year would be preferable to a short-term precision study but is logistically much more difficult to do. The calculation of the precision value is also different, requiring the use of a statistical technique called linear regression, because biological changes would be expected to occur during the longer time frame. Instead of the SD, a different quantity, called the standard error of the estimate, is calculated and used to express precision (3). Because of the longer time involved, the possibility of other errors in the test increases, such as errors from machine drift and differences in operator techniques. Consequently, long-term precision

Table 6-3
Z' Values for Various Levels of Statistical Confidence

Statistical confidence level (%)	Z' value
99	2.58
95	1.96
90	1.65
80	1.28

estimates tend to be poorer than short-term precision estimates. Although a long-term precision study is a more appropriate reflection of the relevant circumstances in clinical practice, the logistical difficulties of performing such a study make it impractical.

DETERMINATION OF LEAST SIGNIFICANT CHANGE

Once the precision of the measurement at any given skeletal site is known, the magnitude of the change in bone density at that site that indicates real biological change can be determined. This is called the least significant change (LSC). To determine the LSC, a decision must be made as to what level of statistical confidence is needed and how many measurements will be done at baseline and follow-up. Ideally, 95% statistical confidence is chosen, but 80% is generally more than adequate for clinical decisions.

The formula for determining the LSC is as follows:

$$LSC = Z'(Pr) \sqrt{\frac{1}{n_1} + \frac{1}{n_2}} \qquad (9)$$

in which Z' (pronounced "Z prime") is the value chosen based on the desired level of statistical confidence, Pr is the precision value as either the RMS-SD or the RMS-CV, n_1 is the number of baseline measurements, and n_2 is the number of follow-up measurements. Z' values are chosen from tables of such values usually found in statistical or mathematical texts. Table 6-3 gives Z' values for various levels of confidence.

For any precision value and any number of baseline and follow-up measurements, the magnitude of the change needed for statistical significance, the LSC, will be less at lower levels of statistical confidence. The magnitude of the LSC can also be reduced for any level of statistical

confidence by increasing the number of measurements performed at baseline and follow-up. In clinical practice, one measurement is commonly
done at baseline and again at follow-up. When 1 is substituted for both
n_1 and n_2 in Eq. 9, the sum under the square root sign becomes 2, as
shown in Eq. 10:

$$LSC = Z'(Pr) \sqrt{\frac{1}{1} + \frac{1}{1}} = Z'(Pr)\sqrt{2} \qquad (10)$$

The situation, then, of one measurement at baseline and one measurement
at follow-up effectively changes Eq. 10 to Eq. 11, used for the calculation
of the $_{1x1}LSC$:

$$_{1x1}LSC = Z'(Pr)1.414 \qquad (11)$$

If two measurements were done at baseline and again at follow-up, the
sum under the square root sign in Eq. 9 becomes 1, as shown in Eq. 12
for the calculation of the $_{2x2}LSC$:

$$_{2x2}LSC = Z'(Pr)\sqrt{\frac{1}{2} + \frac{1}{2}} = Z'(Pr) \sqrt{1} \qquad (12)$$

This effectively changes the equation for the calculation of the $_{2x2}LSC$ to:

$$_{2x2}LSC = Z'(Pr)1 = Z'(Pr) \qquad (13)$$

Thus, for any level of statistical confidence, the magnitude of the LSC
is reduced by performing duplicate measurements at baseline and follow-
up rather than single measurements because the product of the Z' and
precision values is being multiplied by only 1 instead of 1.414. The LSC
is effectively reduced by approximately 30%.

When the Z' values shown in Table 6-3 for 95 and 80% are substituted
in the formulas for the $_{1x1}LSC$ and the $_{2x2}LSC$, the formulas become

$$_{1x1}LSC^{95} = 1.96(Pr)1.414 = 2.77(Pr) \qquad (14)$$

$$_{1x1}LSC^{80} = 1.28(Pr)1.414 = 1.81(Pr) \qquad (15)$$

$$_{2x2}LSC^{95} = 1.96(Pr)1 = 1.96(Pr) \qquad (16)$$

$$_{2x2}LSC^{80} = 1.28(Pr)1 = 1.28(Pr) \qquad (17)$$

For example, if the RMS-SD precision of PA lumbar spine DXA studies
at a facility were determined to be 0.015 g/cm^2, this value would be
substituted in Eq. 14 if 95% confidence was desired and one measurement
was performed both at baseline and follow-up. In that case, the changes
in Eq. 14 are reflected in Eqs. 18 and 19:

$$_{1x1}LSC^{95} = 2.77(Pr) = 2.77(0.015 \text{ g/cm}^2) \tag{18}$$

$$_{1x1}LSC^{95} = 0.042 \text{ g/cm}^2 \tag{19}$$

For 80% confidence, the precision value of 0.015 g/cm^2 is substituted in Eq. 15, resulting in an LSC of 0.027 g/cm^2. The RMS-%CV can be substituted in a similar fashion for the precision value in Eqs. 14 through 17 to give the LSC as a percentage change from baseline for the various levels of confidence and numbers of measurements.

WHEN SHOULD A MEASUREMENT
BE REPEATED IN CLINICAL PRACTICE?

To determine whether a significant change in the bone density has occurred, the follow-up measurement(s) should be done when enough time has passed for the LSC to be achieved. Therefore, once the magnitude of the LSC has been determined, the time required between measurements is calculated as follows:

$$\text{Time interval} = \text{LSC} \div \text{Expected rate of change per year} \tag{20}$$

The expected rate of change per year for the various therapeutic agents or disease states is determined from the available literature. For example, if the average increase in bone density after 1 year of therapy with some agent is 0.03 g/cm^2 and the LSC in Eq. 19 of 0.042 g/cm^2 is used, the time interval required is as follows:

$$\text{Time interval} = \frac{0.042 \text{ g/cm}^2}{0.03 \text{ g/(cm}^2 \cdot \text{year)}} = 1.4 \text{ year} \tag{21}$$

The follow-up measurement should not be made for 1.4 years because it will take at least that long before the LSC can be expected to have occurred. The LSC and expected rate of change can also be given as percentages. To calculate the LSC as a percentage change from baseline, the RMS-%CV value must be used as the precision value rather than the SD.

WHICH SKELETAL SITE SHOULD BE USED
TO MONITOR CHANGES IN BONE DENSITY?

It is clear, then, that the time interval required to see a significant change is not only dependent on the precision at a site but the expected

Table 6-4
Interrelationship Between Precision and Anticipated
Rate of Change in Determining Time Interval to Obtain LSC

Precision (%CV)	Change per year (%)	Time interval (years)
1.0	1	2.77
	3	0.92
	5	0.55
1.5	1	4.16
	3	1.39
	5	0.83
2	1	5.54
	3	1.85
	5	1.11

rate of change at that site as well. Therefore, if the precision at a particular site is excellent but the anticipated rate of change is very slow, the required time interval may be far too long to be acceptable for clinical purposes. Table 6-4 illustrates the interaction between precision and rate of change and the time interval to the LSC at the 95% confidence level (4).

Precision tends to be the best, and therefore the precision values the lowest, at the PA lumbar spine, total hip, proximal radius, and heel. Rates of change tend to be the greatest at the PA lumbar spine. As a result, the PA lumbar spine is generally used for serial measurements to assess therapeutic efficacy of the currently available agents. The best skeletal site for monitoring any particular therapy or disease state is the site that provides the combination of superior precision and the greatest rate of change.

IS THE MEASURED CHANGE
THE ACTUAL CHANGE IN BMD?

Once the baseline and follow-up bone density measurements have been completed and the magnitude and significance of the change in BMD determined, the range within which the true change actually lies can be calculated. Because there is some statistical uncertainty in both the baseline and follow-up measurements, there is also uncertainty in the magnitude of the measured change. For example, if one baseline and one follow-up bone density measurement are performed at a facility where the precision

Table 6-5
Confidence Intervals for Measured Change
in BMD for Different Values of Precision

Confidence level (%)	Precision (%CV)				
	1	*1.25*	*1.5*	*1.75*	*2.0*
95	±2.77	±3.46	±4.16	±4.85	±5.54
90	±2.33	±2.91	±3.50	±4.08	±4.66
80	±1.81	±2.26	±2.72	±3.12	±3.62

for such testing is 1.5%, at the 95% confidence level the $_{1x1}LSC^{95}$ will have been determined to be 4.16%. If the baseline measurement was 0.854 g/cm^2 and the follow-up measurement was 0.905 g/cm^2, the measured change in bone density is 0.051 g/cm^2, or 6%. Because a 6% change clearly exceeds the $_{1x1}LSC^{95}$ of 4.16%, the measured change is statistically significant at the 95% confidence level. One cannot definitely say, however, that there has actually been a 6% change. The 95% confidence interval for the measured change is actually 6% ± 2.77, or 3.23% to 8.7%. Defining this range is certainly less important than recognizing whether the measured change is statistically significant. Table 6-5 lists the confidence intervals for change in BMD for different precision values given as the %CV when one measurement is performed at baseline and again at follow-up *(4)*.

CASE STUDY IN PRECISION

Assume that the precision for PA lumbar spine studies at a bone densitometry facility was previously determined to be 1.5%. This is the RMS-%CV that was calculated from a study of 10 people, each of whom underwent four studies of the PA lumbar spine. Such a precision study provides 30 df. This means that the calculated precision of 1.5%, at a statistical confidence level of 95%, is at worst actually 34% higher than that, or 2.01% ([1.5% x 34%] + 1.5%). At this same facility, the precision for femoral neck bone density studies was established as 2.4%. At 95% confidence, the worst this precision figure might actually be is 3.2%.

Mrs. Jones, who has a recent diagnosis of osteoporosis, has just received a prescription for a potent antiresorptive agent as treatment for osteoporosis. Her physician has requested that she have repeat bone density studies to assess the effectiveness of the therapy. When should Mrs. Jones's bone density studies be repeated?

There are several factors to be considered in answering what would seem to be a straightforward question. First, what magnitude of change in bone density at the PA lumbar spine and femoral neck is expected over the course of a year with the particular agent that has been prescribed for Mrs. Jones? How many measurements will be done at both baseline and follow-up? And, finally, is 80% confidence sufficient or must the physician be ninety-five percent confident that a real change has occurred? Ninety-five percent confidence will require the most stringent criteria, but 80% is often more than sufficient.

Assume that the therapeutic agent in question has been shown to produce an average increase of 5% from baseline in lumbar spine bone density during the first year of treatment. This same agent generally produces a 2% gain in femoral neck bone density during the same period. One measurement of the PA lumbar spine and one of the femoral neck have already been made and no additional baseline measurements are to be taken. The physician intends to perform only one measurement of the PA lumbar spine and femoral neck at the time of follow-up. The physician would like to be 95% confident that a significant change has occurred but asks that you give him a recommendation for 80% confidence as well.

The follow-up measurements to assess therapeutic efficacy should not be made until sufficient time has passed to allow the LSC to occur. Thus, the first calculation to be made is to find the $_{1x1}$LSC for 80% confidence and the $_{1x1}$LSC for 95% confidence for each of the skeletal sites using the precision values that have been previously established. Equations 14 and 15 can be used to find these values by substituting the RMS-%CV precision values of 1.5% for the PA lumbar spine and 2.4% for the femoral neck into each of the equations. For the lumbar spine, the $_{1x1}$LSC^{95} is 4.16% and the $_{1x1}$LSC^{80} is 2.72%. At the femoral neck, the $_{1x1}$LSC^{95} is 6.65% and the $_{1x1}$LSC^{80} is 4.34%. Given the anticipated rate of change from the chosen therapeutic agent, the length of time it will take to equal or exceed any of these values is the earliest time that the follow-up study should be performed.

If the average increase in lumbar spine bone density with this agent is 5% in the first year, then the $_{1x1}$LSC^{95} of 4.16% should be exceed within 1 year. Using Eq. 20, the exact time can be determined to be 0.8 years. The $_{1x1}$LSC^{80} at the lumbar spine can be reached even more quickly, by 0.54 years. At the femoral neck, however, given that the average increase in bone density is 2% in the first year, the $_{1x1}$LSC^{95} of 6.65% would not be reached for 3.33 years. Even the $_{1x1}$LSC^{80} of 4.34% would not be reached for 2.17 years. It would be reasonable, then, to advise repeating only the PA lumbar spine bone density study in 1 year in anticipation of seeing a change in bone density sufficiently great to conclude that a significant change has occurred with 95% statistical confidence. Repeating the proximal femur bone density study in 1 year would not be reasonable since a significant change in bone density would probably not be detected then, given the precision of testing at the femoral neck and the relatively small anticipated change at that site.

One year later, Mrs. Jones returns for her repeat PA spine bone density study. At the time of her original study, her L1–L4 PA lumbar spine bone density study was 0.734 g/cm². On her repeat study, the L1–L4 BMD was 0.760 g/cm². Is this a significant change? For the change to be significant, the LSC must be equaled or exceeded. In this example, the LSC has been given as a percentage, so the percentage increase from baseline for Mrs. Jones must be calculated. To do this, the baseline BMD value is subtracted from the follow-up value. This difference is divided by the baseline value and multiplied by 100 to express it as a percentage. The formula and the practical application are shown in Eqs. 22–24:

$$\% \text{ Change from baseline} = \qquad (22)$$
$$[(\text{Follow-up BMD} - \text{Baseline BMD})/\text{Baseline BMD}] \times 100$$

$$\% \text{ Change from baseline} = \qquad (23)$$
$$[(0.760 \text{ g/cm}^2 - 0.734 \text{ g/cm}^2)/0.734 \text{ g/cm}^2] \times 100$$

$$\% \text{ Change from baseline} = 3.54\% \qquad (24)$$

The percentage change from baseline of 3.54% does not equal or exceed the $_{1x1}\text{LSC}^{95}$ of 4.16%, so the change cannot be said to be significant at the 95% confidence level. It does exceed the $_{1x1}\text{LSC}^{80}$ of 2.72%, however; thus, the change can be said to be significant at the 80% confidence level.

IMPORTANCE OF PRECISION

When properly performed, bone density measurements are the most precise quantitative measurements in use in clinical medicine today. But it should be clear that until precision studies are performed at a facility, the LSC cannot be determined for any level of statistical confidence, making the interpretation of serial studies impossible. Precision studies do not need to be done on a regular basis, but they should be done at least once. They should be repeated if a new technologist begins scanning or if there is major change in equipment. The patients who participate in precision studies to derive the values that will be used clinically should be representative of the patient population that will be subsequently monitored with the technique. If a densitometry facility employs two or more technologists who are equally likely to perform a patient's bone density study on any given day, then the precision study should be performed by all the technologists, since this will be more representative of what is likely to occur in actual practice. It should be anticipated that the precision will not be quite as good as when only one technologist performs all the studies. It is not uncommon for precision studies to be performed with healthy young adults of normal body size and normal bone density. This type of precision study should be done purely to allow the technologist to test his or her skills in positioning and analysis. The precision value that results from such a study should not be used as the representative precision value for the facility, unless that is the type of patient the facility sees.

The manufacturers of bone densitometry equipment have progressively achieved an increasingly greater degree of automation in the analysis of bone density data, leaving less room for any interaction on the part of the technologist that might introduce error in the analysis. However, positioning the patient and careful monitoring of the data acquisition phase of the scan remain solely under the control of the technologist. If not performed correctly and consistently, the potentially superb precision of these techniques will not be achieved.

REFERENCES

1. (1999) Assessment of instrument performance: precision, installation of new equipment and radiation dose, in *The Evaluation of Osteoporosis* (Blake, G. M., Wahner, H. W., Fogelman, I., eds.), Martin Dunitz, London, pp. 147–172.
2. Glüer, C. C., Blake, G., Lu, Y., Blunt, B. A., Jergas, M., Genant, H. K. (1995) Accurate assessment of precision errors: how to measure the reproducibility of bone densitometry techniques. *Osteoporos. Int.* **5,** 262–270.
3. Verheij, L. F., Blokland, J. A. K., Papapoulos, S. E., Zwinderman, A. H., Pauwels, E. K. J. (1992) Optimization of follow-up measurements of bone mass. *J. Nucl. Med.* **33,** 1406–1410.
4. Bonnick, S. L. (1998) The importance of precision, in *Bone Densitometry in Clinical Practice: Application and Interpretation,* Humana, Totowa, NJ, pp. 83–94.

7

Radiation Safety
in X-Ray Densitometry

X-ray densitometers expose patients to extremely small amounts of radiation in comparison to plain X-ray techniques. These amounts are often so small that they are biologically insignificant. Similarly, the technologist operating an X-ray densitometer on a regular basis is extremely unlikely to be exposed to a significant amount of radiation. Nevertheless, no amount of radiation should be considered inconsequential. The principle of "as low as reasonably achievable" (ALARA) should always be given the highest priority in the operation of these devices.

BASICS OF RADIATION

X rays are a form of electromagnetic energy. Other forms of electromagnetic energy are radio and television waves; microwaves; radar; infrared, visible, and ultraviolet light; and gamma (γ) radiation. These types of energies form the electromagnetic spectrum of energy. When energy is released and then transmitted through a substance, it is called *radiation*. The substance through which the radiation has passed is said to have been "irradiated" or "exposed" to radiation. Ionizing radiation is radiation that causes the release of an electron from its orbit around an atom when the radiation passes through the substance containing that atom *(1)*. X rays and γ rays are also forms of ionizing radiation.

Quantities of Radiation

In X-ray densitometry, the technologist must be concerned with the amount of ionizing radiation to which both the patient and technologist are exposed. A review of the terminology describing these quantities is necessary before discussing the potential effects of ionizing radiation on living tissue and the exposure levels produced during various densitometry examinations.

THE CURIE

The most basic unit of radiation is the Curie (Ci). It is used to quantify the amount of a radioactive material, not the radiation emitted by the material. The SI* unit equivalent to the Curie is the Becquerel (Bq). Equation 1 is the formula for converting Curies to Becquerels:

$$\text{Ci } (3.7 \times 10^{10}) = \text{Bq} \tag{1}$$

To use this equation, multiply the number of Curies by 3.7×10^{10} to determine the number of Becquerels. Amounts of radioactive material are often described as being a certain number of milliCuries or even micro-Curies.

THE ROENTGEN

The Roentgen (R), named for Wilhelm Roentgen who discovered X rays, is used to describe a quantity of radiation exposure, but it is only used to describe the interaction of X rays and γ rays with air. The Roentgen is based on the electrical charge created by the liberation of electrons that occurs during ionization. In densitometry, the Roentgen is rarely used

---

*The system of units known as Le Systeme International d'Unites, or SI, and considered the preferred method of expressing scientific quantities.

except to describe measured amounts of scatter radiation in the air when the devices are in use. This quantity is quite low and generally expressed in milliRoentgens (mR). The Roentgen also has an SI counterpart, called the coulomb per kilogram (C/kg). Equation 2 gives the mathematical conversion of Roentgens to coulombs per kilogram:

$$R(2.58 \times 10^{-4}) = C/kg \qquad (2)$$

THE RAD

Both an abbreviation and an acronym, rad means radiation absorbed dose. It is used in conjunction with any kind of ionizing radiation and any type of substance that has been exposed to ionizing radiation. The rad is commonly used to express the quantity of radiation received by a patient. The biological effects of radiation are often associated with various quantities of radiation given as rads. The SI rad equivalent is the Gray (Gy).* The mathematical relationship between the rad and Gy is simple: 100 rad = 1 Gy. This is expressed in Eq. 3.

$$rad(0.01) = Gy \qquad (3)$$

For medical X rays, 1 R is considered to be approximately equal to 1 rad because the radiation exposure to human tissue from 1 R is only about 5% more than 1 rad.

THE REM

Also both an abbreviation and an acronym, rem means rad equivalent man. The rem expresses the quantity of radiation received by a patient, but unlike the rad, the quantity has been adjusted to reflect the type or quality of radiation involved (2). This recognizes that different types of ionizing radiation have different potentials to do harm. Equation 4 expresses the conversion of rads to rems:

$$rem = rad \times quality\ factor \qquad (4)$$

Medical X rays are assigned a quality factor of 1. As a consequence, multiplying the number of rads by a medical X ray quality factor of 1 does not change the value. For medical X rays, then, in the context of whole-body exposure, 1 rad is equal to 1 rem. By extension, for medical

---

*The Gray is named for Louis Gray (1905–1965), one of the creators of the Bragg-Gray Theory used in radiation therapy.

X rays, 1 R is also approximately equal to 1 rem. This is not true for all types of ionizing radiation, however. For example, alpha particle radiation, as seen with radon exposure, has a quality factor of 20. Because radon is a gas, this exposure reflects the dose to the lungs. The exposure from medical X rays in rads or rems is often called the *skin dose*.

The SI equivalent of the rem is the Sievert (Sv).* The mathematical relationship between the rem and Sievert is the same as between the rad and Gray: 100 rems are equal to 1 Sv. This is expressed in Eq. 5:

$$rem(0.01) = Sv \qquad (5)$$

THE EFFECTIVE DOSE EQUIVALENT

The effective dose equivalent (H_E) is a concept, rather than a particular unit of measure. The concept was introduced in 1987 in an attempt to relate the magnitude of an exposure in rems or Sieverts to the *risk created by that exposure (3)*. As noted in the discussion of the rem, the dose in rads must be multiplied by a quality factor for the type of ionizing radiation, recognizing that different types of radiation have different potentials to do harm. Similarly, different tissues or organs within the human body have different sensitivities to radiation, some being more sensitive than others. It matters, then, what tissues are being irradiated in determining what the risk of that irradiation truly is. This is the concept behind the effective dose equivalent. Tissue weighting factors are assigned to the various tissues in the body. The H_E is determined by multiplying the value in rems or Sieverts by the tissue sensitivity weighting factor. Because the tissue weighting factor has no units of its own, the H_E is still expressed in rems or Sieverts.

The body as a whole is assigned a tissue weighting factor of 1. Individual tissues or organs have sensitivity weighting factors <1 and vary widely. The ovaries and testes are assigned one of the highest values at 0.25 *(4)*. The thyroid's sensitivity is relatively low at 0.03. The red bone marrow is assigned a sensitivity weighting factor of 0.12. The H_E that is calculated for the exposure of any given area of the body is an expression of the risk that would result if the *entire body* were exposed to the same amount of radiation. For example, the H_E for a radiographic absorptiometry study of the phalanges on the Metriscan™ is stated as being less than 0.0001 mrem or <0.012 μSv *(5)*. This means that the risk of the radiation exposure

---

§The Sievert is named for a Swedish scientist who was a member of the International Committee on Radiation Protection.

from such a densitometry study of the phalanges is the same as if the entire body were exposed to less than 0.0001 mrem. This is not a measure of the amount of radiation exposure to the phalanges. The H_E is an expression of the biologically important risk associated with any given amount of radiation exposure.

HARMFUL EFFECTS OF IONIZING RADIATION

Ionizing radiation has the potential to harm living tissue. In addition to medical X rays, there are other sources of ionizing radiation. One important source found naturally in the environment is radon. Radon is a gas formed by the decay of uranium, which is normally found in small amounts in the earth. Materials that are derived from the earth, such as concrete and brick, contain small amounts of radon to which everyone is exposed. The largest source of man-made ionizing radiation is medical X rays. Other man-made sources include nuclear power generators, consumer products such as smoke detectors and televisions, and industrial sources. In comparison with natural environmental radiation, man-made sources of ionizing radiation contribute very little to the total annual radiation exposure of an individual. Nevertheless, ionizing radiation does have the potential to be harmful. The decision to expose a patient to ionizing radiation, no matter how small the amount, should not be made lightly.

Although ionizing radiation can increase the expected number of mutations, the mutations that result are not unique. In spite of the frightening and bizarre images seen in movies of giant crickets devouring cities after being exposed to ionizing radiation, the types of mutations that are actually seen are those that occur in nature. They simply will occur more frequently. Similarly, cancers that can result from high doses of ionizing radiation are not unique. The incidence of almost all types of cancer increases after exposure to high doses of ionizing radiation, but these are the same cancers seen in individuals who have not been exposed.

Acute Lethal Radiation Syndromes

Acute lethal radiation syndromes are mentioned here only for the sake of completeness. They cannot occur with the devices used in densitometry, because the radiation doses required to produce them are thousands of times greater than those used in densitometry. Dual-energy X-ray absorptiometry (DXA) and single-energy X-ray absorptiometry (SXA) X-ray tubes are incapable of producing the high doses of radiation necessary to cause these syndromes, because of their relatively low applied voltage and current. The peak kilovoltage (kVp) of the tube determines the amount of radiation that can be delivered by the tube. The X-ray tube current in milliamperes (mA) determines the number of X rays that are produced, which also affects the amount of radiation produced. In densitometry X-ray tubes, the kVp and mA are far too low to cause any of these syndromes. Nevertheless, the technologist should be aware of them, if only to reassure the anxious patient that they *cannot occur* with X-ray densitometry.

There are three different acute syndromes that ultimately result in death: hematologic death, gastrointestinal (GI) death, and central nervous system (CNS) death. Doses of 200 to 1000 rads can cause nausea, vomiting, diarrhea, hemorrhage, and a decrease in the white blood cell count, leading to infection and fever. Hematologic death occurs within 10 to 60 days. Higher doses of 1000 to 5000 rads result in GI death in 4 to 10 days preceded by lethargy and shock as well as all the signs and symptoms seen with the hematologic death syndrome. Doses of more than 5000 rads result in CNS death within 3 days of exposure. Loss of coordination, meningitis, and the signs and symptoms seen in the GI and hematologic syndromes are also present. These types of syndromes were seen in the unfortunate victims of the Chernobyl nuclear power plant accident in 1986.

Local Tissue Damage from Radiation

Any tissue can suffer acute radiation damage if the dose is high enough. Like the acute lethal radiation syndromes, the doses employed in bone densitometry are much too low to cause immediate tissue damage, but it may be necessary for the technologist to reassure the patient that such damage cannot occur.

SKIN

Reddening of the skin, or erythema, can follow a single dose of 300 to 1000 rads. Persons who have undergone radiation therapy for cancer may have experienced erythema in the course of their therapy. The erythema may be followed by a sloughing of the skin, called *desquamation*. The dose that has been determined to cause erythema in about 50% of the persons exposed is 600 rads (6 Gy) *(6)*. This is, again, a dose that is thousands of times higher than the doses given with bone densitometry, and, consequently, erythema of the skin after a bone density study simply cannot occur.

OVARIES AND TESTES

The sensitivity of the ovaries to radiation changes with age. The ovaries are very sensitive in childhood and again after the age of 30 up until menopause. A radiation dose of 10 rads in a mature woman can cause a delay in menstruation *(6)*. A higher dose of 200 rads can cause temporary sterility, and a dose of 500 rads can cause permanent sterility. It is also possible that doses of 25 to 50 rads can produce genetic mutations in the oocytes without killing them such that birth defects could result if fertilization of one of these damaged oocytes were to occur. For this reason, some authorities have recommended delaying attempts at pregnancy for several months after receiving such a dose of radiation.

The testes are also sensitive to radiation. Doses of 10 rads have been reported to cause a decrease in the number of sperm. A dose of 200 rads can produce temporary sterility, and 500 rads can cause permanent sterility. Like the oocytes in the ovary, genetic mutations in surviving sperm are reason to advise men receiving such doses of radiation to avoid attempts at inducing pregnancy for several months.

BONE MARROW AND BLOOD

Irradiation of the bone marrow can cause a drop in the number of red cells, white cells, and platelets. The most sensitive cell appears to be the white blood cell, known as the lymphocyte. Another type of white blood cell, the granulocyte, is less sensitive. The platelets, the small cells responsible for clot initiation, are less sensitive than white blood cells, and the red blood cells are the least sensitive of all. Radiation doses generally in excess of 25 rads are required to see a demonstrable effect on the most sensitive lymphocytes. The effect on the lymphocytes is rapid and recovery is slow. The drop in the number of the other cell types is less rapid and recovery is quicker.

Late Effects of Ionizing Radiation

As a practical matter, the late effects of ionizing radiation are more of a concern to those who work with radiation rather than to patients who undergo an occasional X ray. Although late effects can follow a single high dose of radiation, there is greater concern that they will follow low doses received over a prolonged period, such as might be seen in a radiologic technologist or physician working with an X-ray device. A technologist who works solely with X-ray densitometry, again because of the very low doses employed, will not accumulate sufficient radiation exposure to be at increased risk for these late effects.

The late effect of most concern is cancer. As noted earlier, radiation has been implicated as a cause of almost every type of cancer. Leukemia and thyroid, skin, bone, lung, and liver cancers have been strongly associated with certain types of ionizing radiation. It is difficult to state with certainty the exact amount of radiation that one must receive to be at increased risk for cancer. What does seem clear is that this amount is hundreds or even thousands of times higher than the amount to which a DXA or SXA technologist would be exposed. Even the most basic radiation safety program will reduce the risk further still.

RADIATION DOSES IN DENSITOMETRY

The X-ray tubes used in densitometry devices have kVp and mA characteristics that prohibit the generation of high doses of radiation. The kVp and mA specifications for various devices are listed in the descriptions of the devices in Chapter 4. The technologist should be familiar with the patient doses for the various types of X-ray densitometry studies and how these doses compare to other types of radiation exposure. The point here is not to minimize the importance of any radiation exposure but to put the amount of exposure in perspective to allay unnecessary fears about the exposure.

A certain amount of radiation exposure occurs as a result of sources in the environment. The effective dose from natural background sources is estimated to be 0.6 to 0.7 mrem/day (6 to 7 µSv/day), or about 240 mrem/year (2400 µSv/year) (4). Living at higher altitudes such as a mile above sea level increases this environmental radiation by about 5 mrem/ months (50 µSv/months). A posteroanterior (PA) spine DXA pencil-beam study generally results in an effective dose of only 1 µSv (0.1 mrem). Quantitative computed tomography (QCT) bone density studies do result in slightly higher effective doses than pencil-beam DXA PA spine studies. A QCT spine study may have an effective dose of about 3 mrem (30 µSv). By comparison, the effective dose for an anteroposterior (AP) chest X-ray is about 5 mrem (50 µSv) and for a plain lateral lumbar spine film, about 70 mrem (700 µSv). The radiation doses for various types of densitometry studies, as provided by the manufacturers, are listed in Chapter 4. In some cases, these are the skin doses and in others, the effective dose equivalents.

The kVp and mA of an X-ray tube were noted earlier as determining the amount of radiation produced by the tube. The skin and effective doses seen in bone densitometry studies vary depending on the scan speed and length (7). The dose increases as the scan speed decreases and the scan length increases. On many devices, the technologist can select the mA as well as the scan speed and length. Although decreasing the mA and increasing the scan speed decreases the skin and effective radiation doses, it also tends to reduce the precision of the measurement.§ The effect of increasing scan length on increasing dose, however, makes it even more important that the technologist both perform and recognize a technically good study to avoid repeat starts and excessive scanning.

Multiple bone density studies will also result in greater effective dose equivalents. For example, it is not uncommon for a woman to undergo both a PA spine and proximal femur bone density study on the same day. The total effective dose for that patient is the sum of the effective doses for the individual studies. It also makes a difference whether the woman is pre- or postmenopausal. The effective dose during a DXA proximal femur study will be greater for a premenopausal woman because the effect on the ovaries must be considered. For a postmenopausal woman, the effect on the ovaries need not be considered. Skin doses may be higher in some projections because of higher mA values used in that scan mode, but if the scan length is shorter and important tissues are no longer in the beam path, the effective dose can still be comparable to other projections using lower mA values with resulting lower skin doses.

Fan-array DXA scanners tend to have higher effective doses per scan than pencil-beam scanners.** This is because of higher X-ray tube voltages and currents that are employed in these scanners. For example, the effective dose for a PA lumbar spine study of L1–L4 on a Hologic QDR 1000, a pencil-beam DXA device, is estimated to be 0.05 mrem (0.5 µSv) (8). On a QDR 4500, a fan-array DXA device, this dose may increase to 0.67 mrem (6.7 µSv) (9). Although the effective dose on the fan-array scanner is more than 10 times higher than that for the pencil-beam scanner, it is still no more than the effective dose from natural background radiation for 1 day.

The effective dose during a QCT spine bone density, like that of its DXA counterpart, depends on the kVp and mA. It also depends on the

---

§See Chapter 6 for a discussion of precision in bone densitometry.
**See Chapter 2 for a discussion of pencil-beam versus fan-array DXA scanners.

number of slices made during the study and the thickness of those slices. Usually three slices 8- to 10-mm thick are made. As a consequence, the area that is irradiated is quite small and the effective dose is much lower than might otherwise be anticipated. If a scout scan precedes the actual QCT examination for localization purposes, the effective dose is the sum of the effective doses of the scout scan and the actual QCT study. This total effective dose has been estimated at 6 mrem (60 µSv), but this may be an underestimation *(4,7)*.

Plain lumbar spine films are occasionally obtained either prior to or after DXA spine studies to aid in vertebral identification or the assessment of vertebral deformities. This adds significantly to the effective radiation dose received by the patient. The effective dose from a lateral lumbar spine film alone may be 60 to 70 mrem (600 to 700 µSv). If a lateral thoracic film is obtained as well, the effective dose will be even higher. It is imperative, then, that the technologist learn to identify the vertebrae based on their appearance on the densitometry image, their spatial relationships to other skeletal structures, and the various probabilities of types of segmentation to avoid needing plain spine film solely for the purpose of vertebral labeling.[‡] Morphometry and vertebral imaging without morphometry as performed on some of the newest DXA devices may also reduce the need for plain films in the assessment of vertebral deformities. These types of DXA scans can be performed rapidly with much lower effective doses than plain films of the thoracic or lumbar spine. In addition to the added clinical value of assessing vertebral deformities at the time of the bone density study, the lower effective dose makes these new DXA applications a safer alternative to plain films. The effective dose for vertebral morphometry on a Hologic QDR 4500 has been estimated as 4.1 mrem (41 µSv) in one of the slower scan modes. On the Lunar Expert-XL, the effective dose for vertebral morphometry has been estimated at 3.8 mrem (38 µSv). Both of these doses are considerably lower than the 60 to 70 mrem (600 to 700 µSv) for lateral thoracic and lumbar spine films. Spine imaging without morphometry such as Hologic's single energy Instant Vertebral Assessment™ and GE Lunar's dual energy Lateral Vertebral Assessment™ can be performed at an effective dose less than DXA morphometry and at a fraction of the effective dose for lateral spine films.

[‡]Chapter 3 for a discussion of skeletal anatomy and identification of the vertebrae.

RADIATION PROTECTION PROGRAMS

Radiation protection programs, even in bone densitometry facilities, are based on the premise that any unnecessary radiation exposure is unacceptable, no matter how small. The guiding principle of all such programs is ALARA. There are three aspects to any radiation protection program. One is the protection of the public. Another is the protection of the patient. The final aspect is the protection of the technologists and physicians involved in the operation of radiologic devices. Limits for radiation exposure have been set for members of the public and for radiation workers such as technologists and physicians. *Members of the public* refers to individuals who are not undergoing radiologic procedures and who do not work with radiation-producing devices or substances. These limits have changed over the years to reflect increasing knowledge about the effects of ionizing radiation. A member of the public may receive a dose of 0.1 rem (1 mSv) per year while a radiation worker may receive a dose of 5 rem (50 mSv) per year and still be considered to have exposures within permissible limits *(10)*. The lifetime effective dose limit in rems for a radiation worker should not exceed his or her age in years. Although it is extremely unlikely that a member of the public who is consistently in the vicinity of a DXA device or a radiation worker dealing solely with DXA devices would ever exceed those limits, radiation protection programs can be designed to ensure this.

The exact requirements for any radiation protection program may vary from state to state. It is imperative, therefore, that the state regulations be reviewed to ensure compliance. In facilities in which the only radiologic device is a DXA densitometer, the regulations pertaining to radiation safety are generally minimal. However, even in the absence of any regulations, there are some simple but appropriate measures that should be considered.

Protection of the Public

The first measure is to "post" the room in which the densitometer is kept. *Posting* means placing radiation warning signs on the entrances to the room and restricting access. This is generally a requirement when radiation levels are 5 mrem/hour (50 μSv/hour) or more in the area housing the X-ray device. With most densitometers, radiation levels will not approach this threshold. Nevertheless, it seems reasonable to place warning signs on the entrances and to restrict access. This is simply a matter of

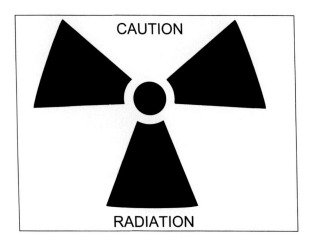

Fig. 7-1. Radiation warning sign. The fan blades are traditionally magenta on a yellow background.

fully informing the public and protecting expensive medical devices. Figure 7-1 shows the traditional X-ray warning sign. The fan blades of the sign are normally magenta on a yellow background. Professionally produced signs are inexpensive and available from a variety of X-ray supply companies.

Consideration should also be given to a radiation survey. A radiation physicist can document readings with a counter in and around the densitometer when the densitometer is in operation. Such readings should be taken at specific distances from the X-ray tube within the room as well as outside of the room. If there are offices or hallways next to the densitometry room that the public has occasion to frequent, readings should be taken there as well. This includes offices on floors both above and below the densitometry room. The readings at each location should be documented in some way and signed and dated by the individual making the readings. It is quite likely that there will be no detectable counts on the counter when this is done. Nevertheless, this documentation can be invaluable in allaying unjustified fears about radiation exposure among members of the public.

Individuals who are not directly involved in performing a bone density test should not be in the densitometry room during testing. This is again an additional safeguard against even the smallest amount of unnecessary radiation exposure. If a radiation survey has been done and no detectable counts have been documented at a specific distance from the X-ray tube, exceptions can be made on a case-by-case basis as long as the individual stays the documented safe distance away from the tube. If a radiation survey has not been done, allowing members of the public in the room is not advisable under any circumstances.

Protection of the Patient

The patient undergoing a bone density study is not technically considered a member of the public for radiation protection purposes. The technologist must assume a major role in protecting these individuals from unnecessary radiation as well. It is not the responsibility of the technologist to order the bone density study; it is the physician's. In a sense, the technologist cannot control the ordering of unnecessary bone density studies. This does not mean, however, that the technologist should abandon all thoughts of what he or she knows to be appropriate once the patient has arrived for testing. The knowledgeable technologist can aid the physician, enhance the care of the patient, and protect the patient from unnecessary radiation exposure without intruding on the physician-patient relationship or undermining the patient's confidence in his or her physician.

Patients should always be asked whether they have had a previous bone density study, and if so, where, when and on what type of machine. It is not uncommon for the patient to have had a bone density study by any technique of the peripheral skeleton that suggests bone loss prompting the physician to request a study of the spine or proximal femur almost immediately. This is appropriate in many circumstances. On the other hand, if the patient is undergoing treatment for bone loss and being followed with bone density measurements, the bone density measurements should ideally be made on the same machine every time. If the same machine is not used, then the next best choice is the same type of machine. If the patient's previous bone density study was at another facility on a different type of machine, it would be in the patient's best interests to return to that facility if possible. A test on another type of machine will not be interpretable in the context of judging a change in bone density rendering that radiation exposure unjustified.

The timing of the repeat study is also important. Rarely are repeat studies justified more often than once a year at the spine and more often than every 2 years at the proximal femur. The most notable exception is patients receiving corticosteroids who may indeed undergo a follow-up spine bone density study after only 6 months. The appropriate timing of the repeat bone density study is determined by the precision of the measurement at the bone density facility at the particular skeletal site in

---

Pregnant?

If you are pregnant, or think you may be, tell the X-ray

technologist before having an X-ray taken

¿Embarazo?

Si usted esta embarazada o cree que lo esta informe al

technologo antes de que le tomen los rayos-X.

Fig. 7-2. Pregnancy warning sign in English and Spanish.

question and by the expected rate of change in the bone density at that site.[#] If the study appears to have been ordered too soon, such that a significant change in bone density is unlikely, it is appropriate for the technologist to confirm the physician's desire to have this test done now. Once again, a test done too soon for the purposes of following therapy is a test that exposes the patient to unnecessary radiation.

It is also incumbent on the technologist to perform every test correctly. This includes the correct choice of scan mode and speed when these attributes are modifiable, correct patient positioning, as well as correct data acquisition and analysis. If it is not possible to position the patient correctly because of some arthritic or disease process, then the particular study should not be done. This is not the fault of the technologist; this is the expertise of the technologist in preventing the performance of an inappropriate bone density study. The physician should simply be notified, the reasons given, and a request made for suggestions as to how to proceed.

Within the area there should also be signs that prompt a woman to disclose a pregnancy or the possibility of pregnancy. The wording for such a sign is shown in Fig. 7-2 in both English and Spanish. In clinical

---

[#]See Chapter 6 for a discussion of issues surrounding precision and the timing of repeat measurements.

medicine, there is little reason if any to perform a bone density study on a woman who is pregnant or might be pregnant. There are simply no emergency bone density studies. Although it has been suggested that the effective doses are so low to the fetus that even asking about pregnancy is not necessary, there is simply no reason to abandon this precautionary measure *(11)*. Do not assume that because the sign is posted on the wall that the patient has read it. Ask the question directly, explaining that the risk is virtually negligible but that the patient's safety is paramount. Another approach to this issue is the "10-day rule," which states that a radiologic examination should only be performed within 10 days of a woman's last menstrual period. In any case, it is far better to err on the side of caution in deciding whether to proceed with the examination. Whenever there is any doubt about the possibility of a pregnancy, the test should be postponed.

Protective aprons, gonadal shields, and thyroid collars, while not routinely used in X-ray densitometry, should be available. On occasion, it becomes clear that no amount of explanation will sufficiently allay a patient's fears about radiation. In that circumstance, a protective apron or shield should be made available to the patient if it will not interfere with the test. It is a simple matter with many of the peripheral X-ray densitometers to allow the patient to wear an apron during the study. An apron should always be used with children, preferably with a thyroid collar. Gonadal shields can generally be used for men undergoing spine and proximal femur bone density studies without compromising either study.

Protection of the Technologist

The technologist who works solely with X-ray bone densitometers is unlikely to ever receive significant exposures. The concept of ALARA applies here as well, however. Protection for a technologist involves three concepts: time, distance, and shielding. Tracking radiation exposure over time is an additional safeguard.

Time, Distance, and Shielding

Longer scan times result in greater exposure, for both the patient and the technologist, for any given exposure rate. While the patient is exposed directly to the X-ray beam, the technologist is only concerned with any potential radiation leakage or scatter radiation. As noted previously, the choice of the correct scan speed for a study is an integral part of radiation protection for the patient. It is also offers protection for the technologist.

Radiation leakage and scatter radiation are very low for X-ray densitometers, if they occur at all. The concept of ALARA demands, however, that the shortest appropriate scan speed be chosen for any particular study. This may not necessarily be the shortest scan speed of which the machine is capable. It should simply be the shortest appropriate scan speed for that particular patient undergoing that particular study.

Shielding and distance can be considered together for X-ray densitometers in the context of the protection of the technologist or physician. Because the leakage and scatter radiation are low to nonexistent for pencil-beam DXA devices, the radiation exposure of a technologist or physician should be well below permissible limits at distances of 3 ft (1 m) or more from the X-ray tube (12). For fan-array devices, this distance increases to about 10 ft (3 m). Ideally, then, the technologist should remain this minimum distance away from the X-ray tube when the machine is in operation. These recommended distances are based on the assumption that the densitometer is being utilized maximally. If studies are infrequent, the potential radiation exposure is greatly reduced. In any case, the technologist should not stand or sit within 3 ft of the X-ray tube when the machine is in operation. If this is not possible, a protective barrier should be utilized. When central DXA devices are considered, it should be recognized that the X-ray tube moves during patient scanning. The position of the tube during the entire scan must be considered in determining the necessary distance from the tube. This movement can also be used to the advantage of the technologist. For example, when the tube is homed to the head of the scan table, the workstation may be an unacceptably short distance from the tube. When the tube is moved into position for a spine or proximal femur study, however, this distance automatically increases. Similarly, additional distance may be obtained by performing right proximal femur studies rather than left.

PERSONNEL-MONITORING DEVICES

Radiation-monitoring devices, often called personnel-monitoring devices, are inexpensive safeguards that allow the technologist to track exposure over a lifetime. A monitoring device does not protect the technologist from exposure, but the record that it provides can be used to ensure that the maximum permissible doses are not exceeded. These devices are generally required when it is anticipated that an individual may receive more than one-fourth of the maximum permissible dose. However, they should be provided to any technologist who requests one even if such exposures are not anticipated. The most common types of devices are film badges and thermoluminescence dosimeters (TLDs).

Film badges have been in use since the mid-1940s, but they are giving way to TLDs. Special radiation dosimetry film is placed in the badge that is then worn for no more than 1 month. Film badges are not as sensitive to small exposures as are TLDs, which makes them less useful for the densitometry technologist. The TLD contains an entirely different material such as lithium fluoride, and it generally can be worn for up to 3 months at a time. Both the film badge and the TLD should be worn with their proper side to the front. Ideally, they should be clipped to the collar, but a chest pocket or waist band is acceptable as long as a protective apron is not being worn.

Film badges and TLDs are obtained from certified laboratories to which they are then sent for analysis. The laboratory provides a report to the facility documenting the exposure of the wearer. A control badge or control TLD is provided with each shipment of new personnel monitors. This control should be kept at a location that is distant from the radiation-producing device. The purpose of the control is to document any radiation exposure during the mailing of the personnel monitors. This purpose is defeated if the control is kept in the room with the radiation-producing device. Film badges and TLDs should not be exposed to extreme heat or high humidity, left in cars, or worn during activities not related to the performance of the technologist's professional duties.

THE PREGNANT TECHNOLOGIST

If the technologist becomes pregnant, specific measures can be taken to ensure the protection of the fetus, even though the risk is extraordinarily low if bone densitometry is the only potential source of occupational exposure. First, the technologist should inform her employer in writing that she is pregnant. A protective apron can be provided that should be worn by the technologist. It is also reasonable to wear a second personnel-monitoring device at waist level under the apron to monitor exposure of the fetus. The maximum permissible dose to the fetus according the 1993 National Council on Radiation Protection and Measurements recommendations is 500 mrem (5 mSv) (10). It is extremely unlikely that a densitometry technologist or physician would even remotely approach this level of exposure to a fetus, but the concept of ALARA should always guide radiation protection efforts.

REFERENCES

1. (1993) Concepts of radiation, in *Radiologic Science for Technologists* (Bushong, S. C.), Mosby, St. Louis, pp. 3–17.
2. (1990) Protection, in *Christensen's Physics of Diagnostic Radiology* (Curry, T. S., Dowdey, J. E., Murry, R. C., eds.), Lea & Febiger, Philadelphia, pp. 372–391.
3. National Council on Radiation Protection and Measurements. (1987) Ionizing radiation exposure of the population of the United States. NCRP Report No. 93. NCRP Publications, Bethesda, MD.
4. Kalendar, W. A. (1992) Effective dose values in bone mineral measurements by photon absorptiometry and computed tomography. *Osteoporos. Int.* **2**, 82–87.
5. Information on file. Alara, 2545 Barrington Court, Hayward, CA 94545.
6. (1993) Early effects of radiation, in *Radiologic Science for Technologists* (Bushong, S. C.), Mosby, St. Louis, pp. 559–576.
7. Njeh, C. R., Fuerst, T., Hans, D., Blake, G. M., Genant, H. K. (1999) Radiation exposure in bone mineral density assessment. *Appl. Radiat. Isot.* **50**, 215–236.
8. Lewis, M. D., Blake, G. M., Fogelman, I. (1994) Patient dose in dual X-ray absorptiometry. *Osteoporos. Int.* **1**, 11–15.
9. Patel, R., Lewis, M. D., Blake, G. M., et al. (1996) New generation DXA scanners increase dose to patient and staff, in *Current Research in Osteoporosis and Bone Mineral Measurement IV*, British Institute of Radiology, London, p. 99.
10. National Council on Radiation Protection and Measurements. (1993) Limitations of exposure to ionizing radiation. NCRP Report No. 116. NCRP Publications, Bethesda, MD.
11. Lloyd, T., Eggli, D. F., Miller, K. L., Eggli, K. D., Dodson, W. C. (1998) Radiation dose from DXA scanning to reproductive tissues of females. *J. Clin. Densitom.* **1**, 379–383.
12. Patel, R., Blake, G. M, Batchelor, S., Fogelman, I. (1996) Occupational dose to the radiographer in dual X-ray absorptiometry: a comparison of pencil-beam and fan-beam systems. *Br. J. Radiol.* **69**, 539–543.

8 Quality Control Procedures

Understanding and performing quality control procedures is a critical responsibility of the bone densitometry technologist. Although much has been written about quality control procedures in densitometry, many articles have been directed at centers that participate in clinical research trials rather than clinical practice. Quality control, while absolutely necessary in clinical research, is no less necessary in clinical practice. The original indications for bone mass measurements from the National Osteoporosis Foundation published in 1988 and the guidelines for the clinical applications of bone densitometry from the International Society for Clinical Densitometry published in 1996 called for strict quality control procedures at clinical sites performing densitometry (1,2). Such procedures are crucial to the generation of accurate and precise bone density data. If quality control is poor or absent, the information provided to the physician may be incorrect. The interpretation made by the physician based on that incorrect information would be in error, and the medical management of the patient may be adversely affected. The patient, therefore, will have undergone the test and been exposed to a small amount of radiation inappropriately. In clinical trials, the results from hundreds or thousands of individuals are usually averaged and conclusions based on the average values. Small errors in machine performance are made insignificant by the averaging of so many results. In clinical practice, this luxury does not exist. Decisions are made based on one measurement from one patient, which means that strict quality control in clinical practice is even more important than in clinical trials. In spite of inherently superb accuracy and precision in today's X-ray densitometers, alterations in the functioning of the machines will occur. Quality control procedures to detect these alterations should be utilized by every clinical site performing densitometry, regardless of the frequency with which measurements are performed.

The quality control procedures used in densitometry were derived from procedures originally developed for quality control in analytical chemistry and industry *(3)*. The adaptation of these procedures for use in bone densitometry is generally credited to Drs. Orwoll and Oviatt *(4)*. The most commonly used methods are control tables, visual inspection of a Shewhart chart, Shewhart rules, and the cumulative sum (CUSUM) chart. All of these methods require that a phantom be scanned to establish a baseline value, and then regularly to establish longitudinal values.

PHANTOMS

Manufacturers of today's X-ray-based bone densitometers provide phantoms for use with their machines. Some phantoms, such as the anthropomorphic Hologic spine phantom, are used with densitometers from other manufacturers. The manufacturer-supplied phantom is often designed with the specific attributes of the manufacturer's machine in mind, making it the preferred phantom to use with that machine. The perfect phantom that could be used on all machines to test all things does not yet exist.

Some, but not all, manufacturers provide two phantoms to be used for different purposes. One phantom may be used for daily quality assurance functions during which the mechanical operation and calibration of the machine are tested. The second phantom may be designed to mimic a region of the skeleton and is used for quality control to detect a shift or drift in bone mineral density (BMD) values.

Phantoms that attempt to replicate a particular region of the skeleton are called *anthropomorphic phantoms.* These phantoms are made of hydroxyapatite or aluminum. While hydroxyapatite is an obvious choice for such a phantom, aluminum is appropriate as well since aluminum behaves very much like bone when X-rayed. The phantom is encased in an epoxy-resin or plastic block or placed within some other type of material to simulate human soft tissue. Water or uncooked rice can be used for this purpose. The perfect anthropomorphic phantom would replicate the size and shape of the bone or bones in question, have varying densities within a single bone or region, contain a range of densities likely to be encountered clinically, and be surrounded by a material that adequately mimics human soft tissue. Replicating the size and shape of the particular bone or bones and having a nonuniform density throughout the bone tests the edge-detection methodology of the particular system. In other words, it tests the machine's ability to distinguish bone from soft tissue. If the phantom bears no resemblance in size or shape to the particular bone or has very sharp, smooth edges, or if the density of the material is uniform within the bone, the edge-detection program will not be adequately tested. If the material surrounding the phantom does not adequately replicate human soft tissue, once again the ability of the machine to determine bone from soft tissue is not maximally tested. To test a system's abilities at various levels of bone density, it is desirable to have a range of bone densities contained within the phantom. At the same time, this range should reflect values that are likely to be encountered in clinical practice for the test to be truly useful.

Most of the manufacturer-supplied phantoms in use today have some of these attributes but generally not all. Which attributes are emphasized by a manufacturer generally depends on those attributes that the manufacturer wishes to test as a part of the routine quality control program for their machine. The development of the European Spine Phantom (ESP) was one attempt to develop a more perfect spine phantom that could be used on all central devices. It was developed independently of any manufacturer under the direction of the Committee d'Actions Concertés-Biomedical Engineering (COMAC-BME) *(5)*. The ESP is a semianthropomorphic phantom. Its three vertebrae are made of hydroxyapatite and vary in density. The vertebrae are encased in a plastic and epoxy-resin material equivalent to about 10% fat. The use of the ESP has generally been restricted to clinical research trials, primarily because of its expense. It was originally hoped that the ESP could be used to standardize BMD on any central bone densitometer, but, unfortunately, this has not been the case.

Most daily quality assurance procedures to detect mechanical failures on today's densitometers are automated. The program will indicate a passing or failing condition. Before outright mechanical failure occurs, however, regular scanning of the quality control phantom and the application of Shewhart charts and rules or CUSUM charts can detect drifts or shifts in machine values that require correction in order to ensure continued accuracy and precision. Abrupt shifts in values are generally easy to detect. Drifts can be more subtle and therefore, more insidious. The confirmed occurrence of either indicates that the machine is OOC or "out of control."

USING THE PHANTOM TO CREATE
CONTROL TABLES AND CHARTS

Manufacturers generally recommend scanning the phantom 10 times on the same day without repositioning the phantom between studies. This is also the procedure often used as part of quality control procedures in longitudinal clinical research trials. Subsequent phantom scans are then performed at least three times a week and on every day that a patient is scanned.

The average value of the 10 phantom scans should be calculated. The values that represent the average value ±1.5% should also be calculated. The average value +1.5% and the average value −1.5% become the upper and lower limits of BMD within which all subsequent measurements of the phantom should fall. These upper and lower limits are called *control limits*. A control table, as shown in Table 8-1, can then be created. The first column lists the date of the phantom scan, and the second column gives the actual BMD value. In the third column, a yes or no entry indicates whether the phantom BMD value fell within the established control limits.

A control graph offers some advantages over the control table. A control graph is created using the same average value from 10 consecutive phantom scans and control limits based on ±1.5% of the average value. The vertical axis, or *y*-axis, of the graph reflects the BMD values in grams/ square centimeter (g/cm²). The horizontal axis, or *x*-axis, reflects time in days. The BMD that corresponds to the 10-phantom average should be indicated by drawing a solid horizontal line across the graph. The values of the upper and lower control limits are similarly indicated by drawing a dashed line across the graph. Subsequent phantom values are easily tracked by plotting the results on the control graph. Such a graph is called a *Shewhart chart*.

Table 8-2 gives the results of 10 scans of the anthropomorphic Hologic spine phantom that were performed on a GE Lunar DPX. The average value for the 10 scans was calculated and found to be 1.182 g/cm². To find the upper and lower control limits, the average value was multiplied by 1.5%. This was determined to be 0.018 g/cm² (1.182 g/cm² × 0.015). Therefore, the range of values within which all subsequent phantom scan values should fall is 1.182 ± 0.018 g/cm² or between 1.164 and 1.200 g/ cm². Figure 8-1 is the Shewhart chart that was created for this set of 10 phantom scans onto which subsequent phantom scan values have been plotted. The phantom BMD values obtained over time from a scanner that is operating perfectly should randomly fall on either side of the 10-

Table 8-1
Control Table

Date	Phantom value (g/cm²)	Within control limits
10/9/2000	1.179	Yes
10/10/2000	1.187	Yes
10/11/2000	1.162	No
10/11/2000	1.170	Yes
10/12/2000	1.184	Yes

Control limits of ±1.5% or 1.164 to 1.2 g/cm² were established based on a 10-phantom average BMD of 1.182 g/cm².

Table 8-2
Ten Hologic Spine Phantom Scans Performed on a Lunar DPX
on Same Day to Establish Baseline Phantom BMD Value for Quality Control

Phantom scan no.	Date	L1–L4 BMD (g/cm²)
1	4/22/00	1.181
2	4/22/00	1.173
3	4/22/00	1.176
4	4/22/00	1.180
5	4/22/00	1.190
6	4/22/00	1.174
7	4/22/00	1.189
8	4/22/00	1.192
9	4/22/00	1.177
10	4/22/00	1.187

The average value for the 10 phantom scans is 1.182 g/cm². The SD is 0.007 g/cm² and 1.5% of the average value is 0.018 g/cm².

phantom BMD average value but remain within the control limit boundaries of ±1.5%. If a value falls outside the boundaries, the phantom scan should be repeated immediately. If it falls outside the boundaries again, or "fails," the manufacturer should be contacted for additional instructions.

A visual inspection of the Shewhart chart can also provide more subtle clues to machine malfunction or a machine going OOC. The pattern of the values should be reviewed to ensure that the values appear to be randomly falling on either side of the average value in addition to being within the control limits. If this randomness appears to be lost, the machine may be drifting. If an imaginary straight line drawn through the center

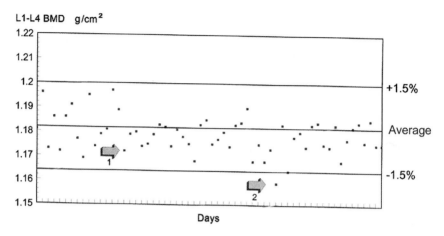

Fig. 8-1. Shewhart control chart. The average BMD of the phantom was established by scanning the phantom 10 times on the same day without repositioning between scans. The control limits were established as ±1.5%. The warning level for application of Shewhart rules was set at ±1.5%. Arrow 1 indicates the point at which it appears that the values are beginning to drift downward, rather than maintaining their random scatter on either side of the average. Arrow 2 indicates the point at which the warning rule was actually violated, triggering the application of the Shewhart rules.

of the phantom values is above or below the average value, a shift may have occurred. In either of these cases, the manufacturer should be contacted for instructions. Inspection of the Shewhart chart in Fig. 8-1 suggests a possible drift in values. Arrow 1 on the graph in Fig. 8-1 indicates a point at which it appears that the phantom values are no longer randomly scattered on either side of the average but instead are concentrated below the average. This suggests that the scan values may be starting to drift downward. These situations can and do occur even though the absolute BMD values obtained from the daily phantom scans remain within the established range and other daily quality assurance procedures continue to give "PASS" indications.

The control table described earlier is simpler to create and maintain than the Shewhart chart, but the ability to visually inspect the data for drifts or shifts is lost. The creation of a Shewhart control table or chart constitutes the minimum quality control program that should be in use in every facility performing densitometry.

The creation of an average baseline phantom value by scanning the phantom 10 times on the same day without repositioning may not reflect the day-to-day variability in machine values and the effects of repositioning that would be expected as the phantom is scanned over time. Consequently,

Table 8-3

Twenty-Five Hologic Spine Phantom Scans Performed on Lunar DPX on 25 Consecutive Days to Establish Baseline Phantom Value for Quality Control

Phantom scan no.	Date	L1–L4 BMD (g/cm²)
1	4/22/00	1.181
2	4/23/00	1.172
3	4/24/00	1.176
4	4/25/00	1.172
5	4/29/00	1.180
6	4/30/00	1.185
7	5/01/00	1.179
8	5/02/00	1.176
9	5/06/00	1.177
10	5/07/00	1.169
11	5/08/00	1.180
12	5/09/00	1.167
13	5/13/00	1.179
14	5/14/00	1.189
15	5/15/00	1.174
16	5/16/00	1.186
17	5/20/00	1.181
18	5/21/00	1.170
19	5/22/00	1.179
20	5/23/00	1.178
21	5/28/00	1.180
22	5/29/00	1.181
23	5/30/00	1.168
24	6/03/00	1.182
25	6/04/00	1.172

The average value for the 25 phantom scans is 1.177 g/cm². The SD is 0.006 g/cm² and 1.5% of the average value is 0.018 g/cm². Compare these average and SD values to those calculated for the 10 scans in Table 8-2.

several groups have recommended that the baseline phantom value be established by scanning the phantom once a day for 25 consecutive days and then averaging these 25 scans. It is thought that this will more accurately reflect the day-to-day variability in machine values and result in fewer "false alarm failures." For example, the average BMD of the same Hologic spine phantom when scanned on 25 consecutive days as shown in Table 8-3 was 1.177 g/cm², resulting in a range for the average ± 1.5% of 1.159 g/cm² to 1.195 g/cm². In both cases, 1.5% of the mean

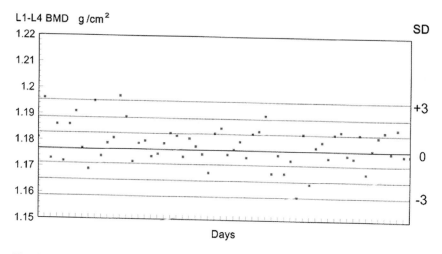

Fig. 8-2. Shewhart control chart. The average BMD of the phantom was established by scanning the phantom once on 25 consecutive days. The values appear to be randomly scattered on either side of the average value. If the warning rule was set at 3 SDs, the application of Shewhart rules would have been triggered on two occasions, seen early in the plot. No other rules were violated, however. As a result, the violations were not confirmed and were considered false alarms.

value was 0.018 g/cm^2, but the range of acceptable values was different from that seen when the phantom was scanned 10 times on the same day without repositioning. Figure 8-2 is a graph of subsequent scans now plotted against the baseline phantom value obtained after scanning the phantom once on each of 25 consecutive days.

Note that in Fig. 8-2, when the mean was calculated using 25 scans performed on consecutive days, the same phantom values do not give any indication of a loss of random scatter. More sophisticated evaluations of this type of data can be done to determine if, in fact, there has been a shift in values. Nevertheless, this type of chart is the foundation of a good quality control program.

METHODS FOR TRACKING MACHINE PERFORMANCE

The field of analytical chemistry recognized the need for strict quality control many years ago. Like bone densitometry, analytical chemistry involves the use of machines for quantitative measurements. Techniques had to be developed to determine that the machines continued to function properly over long periods in order to ensure consistency in the results

(3). The methods common to analytical chemistry have been adapted for use in bone densitometry *(4)*. These methods utilize the BMD values from the phantom scans as described earlier: the average phantom value and the values from phantom scans performed over time. The two most commonly used methods for tracking machine performance are Shewhart rules and the CUSUM chart.

Shewhart Rules

Shewhart rules have been used in analytical chemistry since the 1950s.* To utilize Shewhart rules, it is necessary to establish a baseline value and control limits for the phantom measurement and to create a Shewhart chart as described earlier. In this context, establishment of the baseline value by scanning the phantom once on 25 consecutive days, rather than 10 times on the same day, is recommended, but the 10-phantom average can be used. Once the average value of the 25 phantom scans is determined, the standard deviation (SD) for the set of 25 scans should be calculated. A Shewhart chart can then be created onto which the BMD data from subsequent phantom measurements are plotted, as done in Fig. 8-2. The *y*-axis of the graph should reflect both the actual BMD values and SD units, as shown in Fig. 8-2. To utilize SD units, the average BMD is assigned a value of 0 on the *y*-axis of the graph and the SD tics are labeled +1 or −1, +2 or −2, and so on. In other words, the *y*-axis reflects both the measured BMD and the *z*-score of the daily phantom BMD measurements.** The average phantom value used to construct the Shewhart chart in Fig. 8-2 was previously found to be 1.177 g/cm². The SD was previously found to be 0.006 g/cm² for this set of measurements. It is not necessary to calculate the *z*-score for each of the phantom measurements. When the measured BMD is plotted on the graph, it becomes visually apparent how many SDs from the average the value actually lies because of the SD or *z*-score scale on the y-axis. Remember that with a perfectly functioning

---

*Dr. William Andrew Shewhart (1891–1967), as a scientist with Western Electric, devised the basis for the application of statistical methods to quality control. In 1931, his book, *Economic Control of Quality of Manufactured Product* (D. Van Nostrand, NY), was published, in which he presented his methods for statistical sampling.

**In this context, *z*-score has nothing to do with reference population BMD data. It is simply the number of SDs above or below the average value. See Chapter 1 for a discussion of the *z*-score scale.

machine, the values plotted on the graph are expected to be randomly scattered on either side of the average (i.e., above and below the average).

As these values are being plotted, "rules" are applied to detect trends or "failures" that may indicate a change in machine performance. These are called *Shewhart rules* or *sensitizing rules (6)*. Different combinations of rules have been tested in densitometry in order to minimize false alarms and increase the ability of the Shewhart rules to detect true alterations in machine performance *(4,7,8)*.

Shewhart rules are usually "set" at a certain level. In other words, a triggering or warning level is selected. When this level is exceeded, the Shewhart rules are applied. For example, Shewhart rules may be set at a warning level of the average ± 2 SDs *(3)*. If the phantom BMD value is more than 2 SDs above or below the average BMD, the Shewhart rules are applied to detect potential machine failures.

For example, a machine failure may be deemed to have occurred if the phantom value exceeds the average by ± 2 SDs *and* any one or more of the following Shewhart rules have been violated:

1. A phantom BMD value exceeding the average ± 3 SDs.
2. Two consecutive phantom BMD values on the same side of the average exceeding the average by ± 2SDs.
3. Two consecutive phantom BMD values differing by more than 4 SDs.
4. Four consecutive phantom BMD values on the same side of the average exceeding the average by ± 1SD.
5. Ten consecutive phantom BMD values falling on the same side of the average regardless of their distance from the average.

Not all violations of the rules will be found to be machine failures that require correction and, as such, are considered false alarms. To reduce false alarms, a filter is sometimes applied to the "sensitizing rules." One such filter is to calculate the average BMD for 10 consecutive phantom measurements *after* a violation of one of the Shewhart rules has occurred. If this 10-scan average differs by more than 1 SD from the baseline average value, the violation is confirmed. Another method is to set the triggering of the rules at a higher level, such as the 3 SD deviation level. When this approach is employed, the occurrence of a single value outside the 3 SD limit then triggers the application of the other rules.

Without such filters or triggers, Shewhart rules, although easy to use, produce a high false alarm rate. Even if a machine is in perfect working order, a violation of the Shewhart rules is expected to occur once every 39 scans *(8)*. When the filter is added, the false alarm rate drops to once every 631 scans. Unfortunately, although the addition of the filter to

Shewhart rules reduces the number of false alarms, it may also have the undesirable effect of delaying detection of true shifts in machine performance.

Shewhart rules may also be utilized by calculating the average ± a percentage of the average, as was done in the quality control chart in Fig. 8-1 *(9)*. For most of the central dual-energy X-ray absorptiometry (DXA) scanners in clinical use today, repeat phantom measurements generally result in an SD for the baseline set of phantom measurements that is roughly 0.5% of the average value. Consequently, 1.5% of the average value for the phantom BMD equals approximately 3 SDs. For example, when the statistics were calculated for the 10 phantom measurements performed on the same day shown in Table 8-2, the average was 1.182 g/cm^2 with an SD of 0.007 g/cm^2. One and a half percent of the average was found to be 0.018 g/cm^2. In this case, 1.5% of the average is equal to 2.6 SDs. In the case of the 25 phantom scans shown in Table 8-3 with an SD of 0.006, the 1.5% value of 0.018 g/cm^2 is equal to 3 SDs. The percentage values can be used to invoke the Shewhart rules. Using a value of 0.5% of the average as equaling 1 SD, the Shewhart rules would be applied if a phantom value exceeded the baseline average value ± 1% (instead of the average ± 2 SDs). A violation would be deemed to have occurred under any of the following circumstances:

1. A phantom BMD value exceeds the average by ±1.5%.
2. Two consecutive phantom BMD values on the same side of the average exceed the average by ±1%.
3. Two consecutive phantom BMD values differ by more than 2%.
4. Four consecutive phantom BMD values on the same side of the average exceed the average by ±0.5%.
5. Ten consecutive phantom BMD values fall on the same side of the average regardless of their distance from the average.

The 10-scan average filter described earlier would confirm a failure if the 10-scan average differed from the baseline average by more than 0.5% (instead of 1 SD).

In quality control jargon, each of these rules has its own name. In the order of the previous list, the rules are known as follows:

1. 3 SD or 1.5% rule.
2. 2 SD twice or 1.0% twice rule.
3. Range of 4 SD or range of 2% rule.
4. Four ± 1 SD or Four ± 0.5% rule.
5. Mean × 10 rule.

When any of the Shewhart rules are confirmed, the machine is OOC and the manufacturer should be consulted to determine the cause and corrective action.

CUSUM Charts

CUSUM charts are not as easy to use as Shewhart charts and rules, but these are the types of charts employed by many professional densitometry quality control centers. This technique was originally developed for use in industry and was subsequently adapted for use in bone densitometry *(10)*. The principle underlying CUSUM charts is the expected random variation in the phantom measurement. Remember that even in a perfectly functioning machine, daily phantom BMD values are expected to fall randomly above or below the average phantom value. In other words, the daily phantom BMD value is expected to vary about the average value. The magnitude of the variation, however, even though some measurements will be above (or greater) than the average value and some will be below (or less) than the average value, should remain relatively constant.

To utilize the CUSUM chart, a baseline spine phantom value must again be established by scanning the phantom 10 times consecutively or once on each of 25 consecutive days, as was done previously for the application of Shewhart rules. For all subsequent scans, the difference between the average value and the subsequent value is calculated. The differences are progressively summed and plotted on the CUSUM chart. Mathematically, this is expressed in Eq. 1 as follows:

$$CS_n = \sum_{p=1}^{n}(BMD_p - BMD_{Mean}) \tag{1}$$

in which CS is the cumulative sum and n is the total number of measurements, BMD_{Mean} is the average phantom value, and BMD_p is the phantom value for each of the n measurements. Each sequential value of CS is plotted on the graph. The vertical axis of the graph is marked in SD units of the average value. For a properly functioning machine, the values plotted on the CUSUM chart should be scattered in a horizontal pattern around 0 (0 is equal to the average phantom value). If the pattern is rising or falling, the machine is not functioning properly.

The construction of a CUSUM chart begins again with the data in Table 8-3. The phantom was scanned once each day for 25 consecutive days. The average value of the phantom was found to be 1.177 g/cm², and the SD was calculated to be 0.006 g/cm². Table 8-4 illustrates the calculations of the cumulative sum for the next 10 phantom measurements.

Table 8-4
Calculation of Cumulative Sum for Sequential Phantom Scans

Date	Phantom BMD (g/cm^2)	Difference from average phantom value (g/cm^2)	Cumulative sum of differences (g/cm^2)	Cumulative sum of differences expressed in SD units (z-score)
6/5/96	1.181	0.004	0.004	0.67 (0.004 ÷ 0.006)
6/6/96	1.196	0.019	0.023 (0.004 + 0.019)	4.33 (0.023 ÷ 0.006)
6/10/96	1.173	−0.004	0.019 (0.019 − 0.004)	3.17 (0.019 ÷ 0.006)
6/11/96	1.186	0.009	0.028 (0.019 + 0.009)	4.67 (0.028 ÷ 0.006)
6/12/96	1.172	−0.005	0.023 (0.028 − 0.005)	3.83 (0.023 ÷ 0.006)
6/13/96	1.186	0.009	0.032 (0.023 + 0.009)	5.33 (0.032 ÷ 0.006)
6/17/96	1.191	0.014	0.046 (0.032 + 0.014)	7.66 (0.046 ÷ 0.006)
6/21/96	1.169	−0.008	0.038 (0.046 − 0.008)	6.33 (0.038 ÷ 0.006)
6/24/96	1.195	0.018	0.056 (0.038 − 0.003)	9.33 (0.056 ÷ 0.006)
6/25/96	1.174	−0.003	0.053 (0.056 − 0.003)	8.83 (0.053 ÷ 0.006)

The z-score of the cumulative sum is plotted on the CUSUM chart. The average phantom value is 1.177 g/cm^2 and the SD is 0.006 g/cm^2.

Figure 8-3 illustrates the CUSUM plot for these 10 measurements and 30 additional measurements that followed. In Fig. 8-3, instead of BMD on the vertical axis, SD units or z-scores are utilized. The CUSUM plot for these 40 phantom scans clearly appears to be rising rather than being horizontal.

Although the CUSUM chart is inspected visually to determine machine malfunction indicated by the nonhorizontal plot, two methods have been developed to determine mathematically when control limits have been exceeded. One method involves the superimposition of a V-mask in which the slope of the arms on the mask is determined mathematically (11). The slope is normally some multiple of the standard error of the average phantom value. The stringency of the mask can be changed by increasing or decreasing the slope of the V-mask. The other method, called tabular CUSUM, involves the mathematical calculation of the upper and lower control limits (8). In either case, when values fall outside the control limits or the arms of the mask, an alarm is triggered indicating that the machine is OOC and that the manufacturer should be contacted.

The calculation of the control limits for tabular CUSUM is more tedious than complex, although the equations used for these calculations appear somewhat intimidating at first. The upper control limit is calculated using Eq. 2:

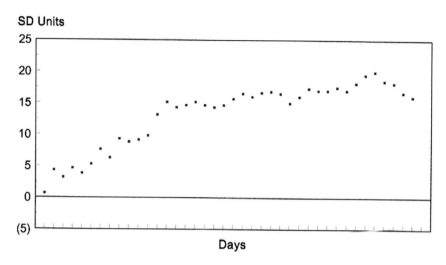

Fig. 8-3. CUSUM quality control plot. The plot clearly appears to be rising, indicating a drift in values.

$$CS_{H_{max}(i)} = \frac{X_i - \mu_0}{\sigma} - k + CS_{H_{max}(i-1)} \tag{2}$$

In other words, to calculate the upper limit of the maximum cumulative sum for scan i $(CS_{H_{max}})$, subtract the average phantom value (μ_0) from the phantom value for scan i (X_i) and then divide this difference by the SD (σ) from the baseline phantom data. Now subtract the value of k, which is taken to be 0.5 (this has the effect of subtracting half an SD). The resulting value is then added to the value of i $(CS_{H_{max}})$ that had been calculated for the previous phantom scan (scan $i - 1$). The lower limit of the maximum cumulative sum is calculated in an analogous fashion using Eq. 3:

$$CS_{L_{max}(i)} = \frac{\mu_0 - X_i}{\sigma} - k + CS_{L_{max}(i-1)} \tag{3}$$

The process is identical except that in this case, the value for phantom scan i is subtracted from the average phantom value, which is the opposite of what was done in order to calculate the upper control limit. When either of the two control limits falls below 0, the CS for that limit is set back to 0, the value that is then used for subsequent calculations for that CS. When either of the CS limits exceeds a value of 5, a possible machine failure is deemed to have occurred. Table 8-5 illustrates the calculation of the upper and lower CS control limits for 10 scans that were performed

Table 8-5
Tabular CUSUM Limits for 10 Phantom Scans Previously Shown in Table 8-4

Date	Phantom BMD (g/cm^2)	$CS_{H_{max}}$	$CS_{L_{max}}$
6/5/00	1.181	0.167	0
6/6/00	1.196	2.834	0
6/10/00	1.173	1.667	0.167
6/11/00	1.186	2.667	0
6/12/00	1.172	1.334	0.333
6/13/00	1.186	2.334	0
6/17/00	1.191	4.167	0
6/21/00	1.169	2.334	0.833
6/24/00	1.195	4.834	0
6/25/00	1.174	3.834	0

The $CS_{H_{max}}$ approached but did not exceed 5. The $CS_{L_{max}}$ was reset to 0 on seven occasions because the value fell below 0. The mean and SD for the baseline phantom values used in these calculations are 1.177 and 0.006 g/cm^2 respectively.

after the initial establishment of the baseline phantom mean value and SD previously shown in Table 8-3.

CUSUM charts or tabular CUSUM are most easily performed with the help of sophisticated statistical software programs. There is no reason, however, that clinical densitometry centers cannot employ CUSUM methodology, even though it is certainly less intuitive to use than Shewhart charts and rules.

AUTOMATED QUALITY CONTROL PROCEDURES

In recent years, densitometry manufacturers have increasingly automated quality control procedures. Calibration standards may be contained within the devices and checked routinely at the touch of a button. Quality control graphs may be generated by the system software, on which phantom values over time are plotted. Shewhart rules may be automatically applied to the results, prompting messages of Pass, Fail, or notification of specific rule failures. Such innovations are indeed welcome, but they are useless unless the technologist performs these procedures on a regular basis. It is also imperative that the technologist knows what to look for and understand the information presented.

Figure 8-4 shows a quality control graph from a Norland XR-Series densitometer. The upper graph reflects the precision of the system *(12)*.

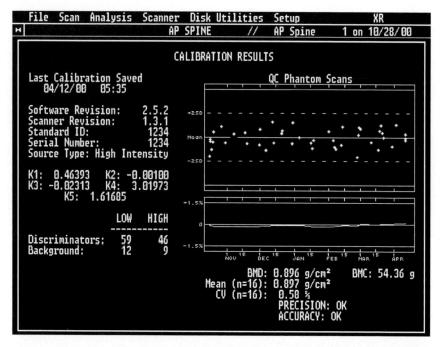

Fig. 8-4. Quality control plot from a Norland XR-series central densitometer. This is a Shewhart chart with control limits of ±2 SDs for precision on the upper graph and ±1.5% for accuracy on the lower graph. The software automatically calculates the average and SD of the last 16 phantom measurements and applies Shewhart rules to determine possible shifts and drifts. The indication of "OK" after accuracy and precision indicates that no rules have been violated.

In this graph, the solid horizontal line reflects the average value for the 16 most recent scans. The dashed horizontal lines indicate ± 2 SDs about the average. The value of the SD used to establish this range is a value for the phantom that is entered into the computer during the setup of the system. The BMD values of the individual scans are plotted on the graph. Approximately 1 of every 20 scans is expected to fall outside the range defined by the average ± 2 SDs simply because statistically this range will contain only 95% of the values. The computer will also calculate the SD for each set of 16 scans. This value is not plotted but is used by the computer. Clearly, the average and SD will change as new phantom scans are performed and added to the set of the 16 most recent scans. This type of calculation is called a *moving average*. The results are monitored for changes in the BMD as well as increases in the SD. Shewhart rules are applied to detect unacceptable changes in the BMD. The acceptable limits for an increase in the SD are calculated mathematically. If the system passes all tests, the notation of "OK" is seen after "PRECISION" at the bottom of the graph. Other messages may be seen, however, which should prompt a call to the manufacturer. For example, an "OUT OF RANGE" notation indicates that the SD from the most recent 16 scans has increased beyond acceptable limits. A "WARNING 1" notation indicates that a single phantom BMD value is more than 3 SDs from the average. This is a violation of the Shewhart 3 SD rule. "WARNING 2" is a violation of either the Shewhart 2 SD twice or Range of 4 SD rule, and "WARNING 3" is a violation of the Shewhart 4 ± 1 SD rule.

The lower graph in Fig. 8.4 reflects the accuracy of the system (12). The middle horizontal line represents the phantom BMD value that was entered into the computer during the setup of the system. The upper and lower horizontal lines indicate a range of ±1.5% about this value. The values plotted on this graph are the average BMD values for the last 16 phantom scans. If the average value for the 16 most recent phantom scans falls within ±1.5% of the true phantom value, "OK" will be seen next to "ACCURACY" at the bottom of the graph. An "OUT OF RANGE" message will appear if the value falls outside those limits. If eight consecutive values fall on the same side of the true phantom value, a "TREND WARNING" message will appear.

The quality control graphs and calculations for the Norland pDEXA® are very similar to those of the XR-Series. The control limits for the accuracy of the pDEXA system are ±2.5% instead of 1.5% (13).

Hologic scanners also provide automated quality control graphing procedures (14). The BMD of a phantom is established during the initial calibration procedures for the scanner. The control limits of ±1.5% of the phantom BMD value are defined on a graph onto which subsequent spine phantom BMD data are plotted. Underneath the graph, two tables are displayed. The table titled "Reference Values" lists the average or mean value and SD for the spine phantom established during machine calibration. The table titled "Plot Statistics" lists the number of phantom scans plotted (n), the mean, the SD, and the percentage coefficient of variation for those scans. There are no sensitizing rules built into the quality control program in the computer. With this automated plot, however, Shewhart rules are easy to apply.

Other manufacturers have automated charting of phantom values. Figure 8-5 is such a chart from the DexaCare Osteometer DTX-200, a dedicated DXA forearm scanner. The dotted horizontal lines on the graph represent control limits of ±1.5%. None of the 85 phantom values has

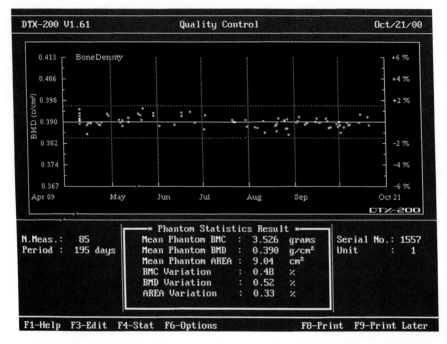

Fig. 8-5. Quality control plot from a DexaCare DTX-200 peripheral densitometer. This is a Shewhart chart with control limits of ±1.5%.

fallen outside the control limits, and the values appear to be randomly scattered about the average value.

If such charts are not available, they are easily created using the information in this chapter. All densitometry centers should implement quality control procedures that minimally consist of control tables or charts with defined control limits of ±1.5% for the average of 10 phantom scans performed on 1 day or 25 scans performed on consecutive days. Shewhart rules with a filter can then be implemented, using rules defined on the basis of percentage or SD, to further strengthen the quality control program. The application of CUSUM charts and calculations as performed at professional quality control centers is more labor-intensive and not necessarily of greater benefit to the clinical densitometry center.

REFERENCES

1. Johnston, C. C., Melton, L. J., Lindsay, R., Eddy, D. M. (1989) Clinical indications for bone mass measurements: a report from the scientific advisory board of the National Osteoporosis Foundation. *J. Bone Miner. Res.* **4,** S1–S28.

2. Miller, P. D., Bonnick, S. L., Rosen, C. J. (1996) Consensus of an international panel on the clinical utility of bone mass measurements in the detection of low bone mass in the adult population. *Calcif. Tissue Int.* **58**, 207–214.

3. Westgard, J. O., Barry, P. L., Hunt, M. R., Groth, T. (1981) A multirule Shewhart Chart for quality control in clinical chemistry. *Clin. Chem.* **27**, 493–501.

4. Orwoll, E. S., Oviatt, S. K., and the Nafarelin Bone Study Group. (1991) Longitudinal precision of dual-energy X-ray absorptiometry in a multicenter trial. *J. Bone Miner. Res.* **6**, 191–197.

5. Kalender, W., Felsenberg, D., Genant, H. K., Fischer, M., Dequeker, J., Reeve, J. (1995) The European spine phantom—a tool for standardization and quality control in spine bone mineral measurements by DXA and QCT. *Eur. J. Radiol.* **20**, 83–92.

6. Montgomery, D.C. (1992) *Introduction to Statistical Quality Control*, Wiley, New York.

7. Orwoll, E. S., Oviatt, S. K., Biddle, J. A. (1993) Precision of dual-energy X-ray absorptiometry: development of quality control rules and their application in longitudinal studies. *J. Bone Miner. Res.* **8**, 693–699.

8. Lu, Y., Mathur, A. K., Blunt, B. A., et al. (1998) Dual X-ray absorptiometry quality control: comparison of visual examination and process-control charts. *J. Bone Miner. Res.* **11**, 626–637.

9. Faulkner, K. G., Glüer, C., Estilo, M., Genant, H. K. (1993) Cross-calibration of DXA equipment: upgrading from a Hologic QDR 1000/W to a QDR 2000. *Calcif. Tissue Int.* **52**, 79–84.

10. (1980) *BS5703: Guide to Data Analysis and Quality Control Using Cusum Techniques*, British Standards Institution, London.

11. Pearson, D. and Cawte, S. A. (1997) Long-term quality control of DXA: a comparison of Shewhart rules and CUSUM charts. *Osteoporos. Int.* **7**, 338–343.

12. (1993) *XR-Series X-Ray Bone Densitometer Operator's Guide*, Norland Medical Systems, Ft. Atkinson, WI.

13. (1996) *Model pDEXA Forearm X-Ray Bone Densitometer Operator's Guide*. Norland Medical Systems, Ft. Atkinson, WI.

14. *QDR 4500 X-Ray Bone Densitometer User's Guide*, Hologic, Waltham, MA.

9 An Overview of Osteoporosis

Osteoporosis is not the only disease process in which bone densitometry is used in diagnosis and management. However, osteoporosis is perhaps the most important disease in which this technology is used, from the standpoint of the prevalence of the disease itself and the number of individuals referred for testing in the context of osteoporosis. It is not the responsibility of the technologist to discuss disease processes with patients referred for testing. In fact, some physicians would consider this intrusive

221

and inappropriate. Nevertheless, the setting in which densitometry is usually performed and the interaction between the technologist and patient is conducive to patients asking the technologist questions about osteoporosis. In these circumstances, it would be inappropriate for a technologist to fail to respond within reason or appear to be uninformed and certainly counterproductive to the technologist-patient relationship. A knowledge of the disease process and the approved therapies for osteoporosis should be part of the densitometry technologist's education. In any discussion with patients, however, it should also be emphasized that the patient's physician is the final authority on the interpretation of bone density results and the need for prescription or nonprescription interventions to prevent or treat osteoporosis.

DEFINITION OF OSTEOPOROSIS

The 1991 and 1993 Consensus Development Conferences

The most widely accepted formal definition of osteoporosis was originally proposed in 1991 and reaffirmed in 1993 at consensus development conferences sponsored by the National Osteoporosis Foundation, European Foundation for Osteoporosis and Bone Disease, and the National Institute of Arthritis and Musculoskeletal and Skin Diseases. At those conferences, osteoporosis was defined as "a systemic skeletal disease, characterized by low bone mass and microarchitectural deterioration of bone tissue with a consequent increase in bone fragility and susceptibility to fracture" (1,2). This definition of osteoporosis was a departure, in many respects, from previous definitions of the disease. Prior to 1991, osteoporosis was often described as an "age-related" disorder, which implied that the inevitability of advancing age alone was reason to develop the disease. This also implied an inability to prevent or even successfully treat osteoporosis. In the 1991 and 1993 consensus conference definitions, there is no longer any mention of aging as a causative factor.

Some definitions of osteoporosis also required that a fracture be present before the disease could be said to exist. The 1991 and 1993 consensus conference definition does not require the presence of a fracture. The definition requires only that the skeleton be sufficiently fragile that an individual is at increased risk for fracture. This approach separates the undesirable outcome of a fragile skeleton—fracture—from the disease process itself. This is similar to the approaches taken with hypertension and hypercholesterolemia. For example, the disease hypertension is based on the finding of increased blood pressure, a quantity that is measured clinically. Once the blood pressure exceeds a certain limit, hypertension is said to exist. Having hypertension places the individual at increased risk for a stroke, although hypertension is not the only cause of stroke. The undesirable outcome of hypertension, then, is a cerebrovascular accident or stoke. The presence of a stroke, however, is not required before it can be said that the disease hypertension exists. The same is true with hypercholesterolemia. This diagnosis is based on the finding of increased levels of cholesterol in the blood, a quantity that is measured clinically. The undesirable outcome of hypercholesterolemia is myocardial infarction or heart attack. However, it is not necessary for a heart attack to have occurred before the diagnosis of hypercholesterolemia is made.

Hypertension and hypercholesterolemia are both diseases that are based on finding abnormal values of quantities that can be measured clinically: blood pressure and cholesterol. Like the definitions of these diseases, the 1991 and 1993 consensus conference definition of osteoporosis suggested that osteoporosis could, at least in part, be defined on the basis of a quantity that could be measured such as the bone mass or density. The clinical measurement of microarchitectural deterioration of bone tissue remains difficult even today. However, the bone mass or density can be readily measured by any one of several different techniques. To complete a clinically useful definition of osteoporosis, the level of bone density that resulted in an increased risk for fracture remained to be determined.

The 1994 World Health Organization Criteria for Diagnosis of Osteoporosis

The World Health Organization (WHO) criteria for the diagnosis of osteoporosis based on the measurement of bone density were published in 1994 (3). At the time the criteria were developed, the WHO was attempting to devise criteria that would allow them to estimate the prevalence or percentage of individuals in different countries who might have osteoporosis. To do this, some common objective definition of osteoporosis was required. The WHO was actually not attempting to specify a level of bone density that would be used clinically in individuals to diagnose osteoporosis.

The levels of bone density that were ultimately chosen by the WHO were based on reviewing the medical literature that was available at the time. After considering several different approaches to establishing the level of bone density that would be called osteoporosis, the WHO stated that a bone mass or bone density that was 2.5 standard deviations (SDs)

Table 9-1
The World Health Organization Criteria for Diagnosis
of Osteoporosis Based on Measurement of Bone Density

Diagnosis	Bone density criteria	T-score criteria
Normal	Not more than 1 SD below the average peak young adult value	Better than or equal to −1
Osteopenia (low bone mass)	More than 1 but not yet 2.5 SDs below the average peak young adult value	Poorer than −1 but better than −2.5
Osteoporosis	2.5 SDs or more below the average peak young adult value	−2.5 or poorer
Severe (established) osteoporosis	2.5 SDs or more below the average peak young adult value + a fracture	−2.5 or poorer + a fracture

or more below the average peak bone mass or density of the young adult was sufficiently low to be called osteoporosis *(3).** This was based on the finding that the percentage of women in the United States and Great Britain who were thought to have a bone density this low at the hip or at the hip, spine, and forearm combined was very similar to the lifetime risk of hip fracture and the lifetime global fracture risk.† The bone mass or bone density was considered normal if it was not more than 1 SD below the average peak bone density of the young adult. Bone mineral densities (BMDs) that were more than 1 but less than 2.5 SDs below the average young adult value were called osteopenic. A fourth category, called severe or established osteoporosis, referred to individuals who had bone densities that were 2.5 SDs or more below the average for a young adult and who also had a fracture. These criteria are summarized in Table 9-1 and again in Appendix II for easy reference. The WHO did not restrict

---

*A standard deviation (SD) is a measure of variability about an average value. See Chapter 6 for a discussion of the mathematical definition of an SD.

†Global fracture risk refers to the risk of developing any and all types of fractures rather than any one type of fracture.

the application of these criteria to measurements at any particular skeletal site while noting that measurements at different sites could result in different diagnoses. The original WHO criteria were given as the number of SDs below the average peak bone mass or density for each diagnostic category. These criteria can readily be converted to T-scores, as shown in Table 9-1, since the definition of the T-score in bone densitometry indicates the number of SDs above or below the average peak bone mass or density.[‡]

The WHO criteria were based on information that was relevant only to Caucasian women. Strictly speaking, then, the WHO criteria should be applied only to Caucasian women. In addition, they are relevant only to postmenopausal Caucasian women. They should not be applied to premenopausal women of any race or ethnicity. The WHO did note in 1994 that in the absence of other criteria, it might not be inappropriate to apply the WHO criteria to mature Caucasian men. Note, again, that the WHO was not attempting to establish diagnostic criteria for the clinician to use in diagnosing individual patients. With the increasing use of bone densitometry, however, and the consensus conference definitions of osteoporosis that included a finding of low bone mass without an objective level being specified, clinicians understandably began to apply the WHO criteria to individual patients. The restriction of the criteria to Caucasian women, however, left the clinician ill prepared to interpret bone density results in women of other races. This dilemma remains unresolved. It is not clear whether different criteria should exist for men as opposed to women and for different races. There is little disagreement that the criteria should not be applied to otherwise healthy children, adolescents, and young adults of either sex or any race.

PREVALENCE OF OSTEOPOROSIS

Prevalence is a statistical term that is best understood as an expression of how common a disease is in any population. Prevalence is often expressed as a percentage. How many people or what percentage of a population would ultimately be said to have osteoporosis? This was actually the question that originally concerned the WHO. The answer clearly depended on what level of bone density was chosen as the diagnostic

---

[‡]See Chapter 1 for a discussion of the T-score and other standard score scales.

threshold for osteoporosis. It could also depend on which skeletal site or combination of sites is measured.

In 1992, it was estimated that 45% of Caucasian women in the United States age 50 and older had osteoporosis if osteoporosis was defined as a bone density more than 2 SDs below the average peak bone density at the spine, hip, or forearm (4). If the skeletal sites were considered separately, 32% would have osteoporosis at the spine, 29% at the hip, and 26% at the forearm. After the publication of the 1994 WHO criteria, in which osteoporosis was defined as a bone density 2.5 SDs or more below the average peak bone density, these estimates were revised (5). Approximately 30% of postmenopausal Caucasian women in the United States were now estimated to have osteoporosis at the spine, hip, or forearm, and 54% were estimated to have osteopenia. When the numbers of postmenopausal Caucasian women with osteopenia and osteoporosis were combined, the number of postmenopausal Caucasian women at risk for fracture was estimated to be 26 million.

Being at risk for fracture does not guarantee that a woman will experience a fracture. The risks, however, are substantial. When all types of osteoporotic fractures are considered, one of every two Caucasian women is expected to experience an osteoporotic fracture in her lifetime (6). The lifetime risk of hip fracture for a Caucasian woman age 50 is 17.5% (4). The lifetime risk for a clinical spine fracture is 15.6%. The risk for a morphometric spine fracture is almost certainly much higher but more difficult to estimate.* Some estimates place this risk as high as 35% (6).

Not surprisingly, the number of osteoporotic fractures that occur each year in the United States is staggering. More than 1 million fractures are attributed to osteoporosis every year. Spine fractures account for more than 500,000 fractures, and hip fractures account for more than 250,000 fractures. In 1995, the total cost of treating these fractures was estimated to be $13.8 billion (7). Costs associated with hip fracture accounted for 63.1% of the total.

CONSEQUENCES OF OSTEOPOROSIS

The consequences of osteoporosis are not restricted to the immediate pain caused by the fracture. Multiple spinal compression fractures lead

---

*A clinical spine fracture is a fracture of the spine that causes symptoms. A morphometric spine fracture is a fracture that is diagnosed on the basis of changes seen on X ray without accompanying symptoms.

to a permanent change in the curvature of the spine known as kyphosis. This spinal curvature is commonly called a widow's hump or dowager's hump. Loss of height also results from compression fractures of the spine. As more height is lost and kyphosis increases, the function of the lungs and gastrointestinal tract is compromised because the organs are being compressed. This can result in a restrictive lung defect leading to shortness of breath (8). The compression of the intestinal tract can lead to early satiety and weight loss. Patients become undernourished, frail, and depressed. The change in the curvature of the spine also results in abnormal mechanical stress being placed on the musculature of the back, causing chronic back pain. Quality of life is greatly diminished.

The consequences of hip fracture are equally if not more devastating. The treatment of hip fracture generally involves surgery, with its attendant morbidity and mortality. It is estimated that one-half of the women who experience hip fracture cannot walk independently 1 year after the fracture. As many as 60% cannot perform the activities of daily living that they could before the fracture (9). This leads to a loss of independence, which can result in referral to a nursing home environment. An excess mortality of up to 20% has been associated with osteoporotic hip fractures (10).*

RISK FACTORS FOR OSTEOPOROSIS

The factors that increase the risk for bone loss or osteoporotic fracture are numerous. These factors either can inhibit the development of a normal peak bone density as a young adult or can cause bone loss after the attainment of peak bone mass. Some factors can affect both.

Attainment of Peak Bone Density

Peak bone density refers to the maximum bone mass or density that is attained in life.† It is the average peak bone density at any given skeletal site that is used as the reference for the T-score. The average age at which peak bone density is reached is the subject of some controversy. It is

---

*Excess mortality refers to the number or percentage of deaths that occur over and above that expected for any given age group.

†The terms *peak bone density* and *peak bone mass* are used interchangeably in this context. This value is also called the *average young-adult bone mass or density.*

likely that the age differs depending on the skeletal site being considered. There is little disagreement that peak bone density is reached by age 35. The disagreement begins as that age is revised downward. Many authorities believe that peak bone density is reached in the spine and proximal femur by age 20 (11–13). Anything that interferes with the development of peak bone density places the individual at greater risk of osteoporosis, because any bone loss that might occur after the attainment of peak bone density will begin from a lower level. There is no question that genetics plays an important role in the maximum level of bone density that is achieved, but perhaps 20% of the determinants of peak bone density are not genetically related. Dietary calcium deficiency and lack of exercise are two factors that have been implicated in the failure to achieve an average peak bone density (14,15).

Maintenance of Bone Density

Once peak bone density has been reached, the density of the skeleton is maintained by the coordinated efforts of the bone-remodeling cells: the osteoblast and osteoclast. The osteoclast actually initiates the resorption or removal of old bone. The osteoblast forms new bone to replace the old bone that has been removed by the osteoclast. In the adult, after the attainment of peak bone density, these processes are balanced or coupled. The amount of bone removed by the osteoclast is replaced by the same amount under the direction of the osteoblast. When these actions are no longer balanced or become uncoupled, bone loss will begin, because excessive bone is being resorbed by the osteoclast, or too little bone is being replaced by the osteoblast, or both.

Bone loss tends to occur with advancing age. Consequently, the term *age-related bone loss* is often used to describe the bone loss that occurs in the absence of an obvious disease process. This bone loss should not be mistakenly considered either normal or desirable. It is also quite likely that as more is learned about the factors that cause bone loss, less will be attributed to age alone. The list of known factors that can cause either an increase in osteoclastic bone resorption or decrease in osteoblastic bone formation is lengthy. Such factors include calcium deficiency; smoking; estrogen deficiency; testosterone deficiency; Cushing's disease; hyperthyroidism; insulin-dependent diabetes; alcohol abuse; malabsorption; and the use of corticosteroids, anticonvulsants, lithium, GnRH agonists, and long-term heparin.

When the bone density is sufficiently low, little provocation is required to cause a fracture. In the spine, coughing, sneezing, or maintaining a flexed posture can cause fractures. Most hip fractures occur after a fall, although most falls are from a standing height or less *(16)*. Any factor that increases the risk of falling can increase the risk of hip fracture. Such factors include poor eyesight, poor balance, muscle weakness, seizure disorders, postural hypotension, and the use of sedating medications.

The risk of osteoporotic fractures is not the same in men and women or among different races. The reasons for this are not entirely clear. There may be genetic differences that result in the attainment of greater or lesser values for peak bone density. Factors that can cause bone loss may be more prevalent in some populations and geographic areas than others. Women have a higher risk of osteoporotic fracture than do men. This is almost certainly attributable, in large part, to estrogen-deficient bone loss that occurs at menopause. Caucasians, as a race, have the highest risk of osteoporotic fracture, whereas African Americans have the lowest *(16)*.

THE NATIONAL OSTEOPOROSIS FOUNDATION GUIDELINES FOR BONE MASS MEASUREMENTS

In 1998, the National Osteoporosis Foundation (NOF) issued guidelines for physicians to help determine which patients should undergo bone density testing *(17)*. These recommendations should not supersede the judgment of physicians regarding the care of individual patients. They are extremely useful, however, in ensuring that the women who should undergo measurement are referred for a measurement. The guidelines were written after a lengthy process involving consultation with many experts and extensive reviews of the medical literature. The majority of the literature available for review dealt with findings in postmenopausal Caucasian women. Like the WHO criteria, because these guidelines were based on information obtained in postmenopausal Caucasian women, they were primarily intended for postmenopausal Caucasian women and not women of other races. Nevertheless, it is not uncommon or considered inappropriate for physicians to utilize these guidelines in the care of women of other races.

Table 9-2 summarizes the NOF guidelines. The list of risk factors that may be considered in determining whether a woman under age 65 should have a measurement is extensive. It is so extensive, in fact, that it is unusual to find a woman who does not have at least one risk factor. Recommending testing women who had been on hormone replacement therapy for prolonged periods was a departure from earlier recommendations. In the past, it was generally assumed that these women were pro-

Table 9-2
The National Osteoporosis Foundation
Recommendations for Bone Mass Measurement Testing

1. Postmenopausal women under age 65 with one or more risk factors other than being postmenopausal.
2. All women age 65 and over. Consideration of other risk factors is not necessary.
3. Postmenopausal women who present with fractures.
4. Women in whom knowledge of their BMD would influence their decision to begin treatment for osteoporosis.
5. Women who have been on hormone replacement therapy for long periods.

tected from bone loss and less likely to obtain useful information from a bone density study. It has become clear, however, that many of these women do have low bone density in spite of prolonged use of hormone replacement therapy such that knowledge of their bone density is useful in optimizing their medical care. In making this recommendation, the NOF was attempting to ensure that these women were not arbitrarily and inappropriately excluded from testing.

THE 1997 BONE MASS MEASUREMENT ACT

The cost of a bone density test has generally fallen over the last 5 years as the devices have become more numerous and widespread. Nevertheless, the cost of testing can deter a woman from undergoing the measurement in some circumstances. In 1998, the Health Care Financing Administration (HCFA) proposed regulations for Medicare coverage of bone mass measurements based on the passage of the 1997 Bone Mass Measurement Act by Congress (18). These regulations went into effect in July 1998. There were five circumstances described in which Medicare would potentially cover the bone mass measurement; Table 9-3 summarizes these. Note that four of the five circumstances refer to an "individual" rather than a "woman." This means, of course, that men as well as women should be covered. Prior to late 2000, there were no treatments for osteoporosis in men approved by the Food and Drug Administration (FDA), so coverage for monitoring therapy was limited to women. In late 2000, alendronate was approved for the treatment of osteoporosis in men so that Medicare should now cover men in this circumstance as well.

Table 9-3
Medicare Coverage for Bone Mass Measurements

---

1. A woman who has been determined by her treating physician or treating qualified nonphysician practitioner to be estrogen deficient and at clinical risk for osteoporosis, based on her medical history and other findings
2. An individual with vertebral abnormalities on X ray suggestive of osteoporosis, osteopenia, or fracture
3. An individual receiving or expected to receive glucocorticoid therapy equivalent to 7.5 mg of prednisone or greater per day for more than 3 months
4. An individual with primary hyperparathyroidism
5. An individual being monitored to assess the response to or efficacy of an FDA-approved drug therapy for osteoporosis

---

Medicare will cover a bone density measurement at one skeletal site by one technique every 23 months. Two exceptions to this "frequency" limitation were specifically noted by HCFA. The first exception was in patients on glucocorticoid therapy for more than 3 months. In this situation, the bone mass measurement could be repeated sooner than 23 months to monitor the bone density. The second exception was when the bone density measurement that led to the initiation of treatment was made with a technique that would not be used for monitoring. In this case, a second bone mass measurement could be made quickly with the monitoring technique in order to establish the baseline for monitoring. HCFA did not exclude the possibility that coverage might be allowed for more frequent measurements in other circumstances, but these were the only two exceptions actually noted in the *Federal Register*. The covered circumstances described by Medicare do not have specific ICD-9 codes.* Several different ICD-9 codes are potentially applicable to each circumstance. Which code a Medicare carrier accepts as justifying coverage can vary from state to state. HCFA has approved the use of a combination of two ICD-9 codes to indicate "an estrogen-deficient woman at clinical risk for osteoporosis." The codes are V82.81, which is the code for special screening for osteoporosis, and V49.81, which is the status code for postmenopausal women. The CPT codes* necessary for billing Medicare for various types of bone density testing are listed in Appendix V.

---

*ICD-9 (International Classification of Disease 9) codes are diagnostic codes used to justify the performance of procedures.
*CPT (Current Procedural Terminology) codes are codes used to identify procedures.

THE NATIONAL OSTEOPOROSIS FOUNDATION GUIDELINES FOR TREATMENT BASED ON BMD TESTING

The NOF also published guidelines for prescription intervention to prevent or treat osteoporosis based on the bone density measurement *(17)*. It was emphasized that women over age 70 with multiple risk factors did not necessarily need a bone density measurement before therapy was initiated. The recommendations for prescription intervention based on the bone density measurement utilize the T-score. The NOF recommended that therapy be initiated in women with T-scores poorer than −2 even if no other risk factors were known to exist. In women with T-scores poorer than −1.5 and at least one other risk factor, the NOF also recommended that prescription intervention be considered. These intervention thresholds suggested by the NOF do not correspond with the diagnostic thresholds suggested by WHO. Even though the diagnostic threshold for osteoporosis as proposed by WHO was set at a T-score of −2.5, the risk of fracture is present at higher levels of bone density. The NOF intervention thresholds recognize this, and, consequently, intervention is recommended at T-scores of −1.5 or −2.0, depending on the presence of other risk factors.

INTERVENTIONS IN OSTEOPOROSIS

Interventions in osteoporosis are divided into two basic categories: nonprescription and prescription. The nonprescription interventions can be further divided into lifestyle modifications and over-the-counter supplements or medications.

Nonprescription Interventions

LIFESTYLE MODIFICATIONS

Many lifestyle modifications recommended to prevent bone loss and fractures are appropriate for everyone in general, not just the woman concerned about osteoporosis. In some cases, however, the recommendations are different if the woman already has a very low bone density or fracture compared with the woman who has a normal bone density and is concerned about future bone loss. Recommendations that are appropriate for everyone include the following:

1. Avoidance of cigarette smoke
2. Moderation in alcohol intake

Table 9-4
1994 National Institutes of Health (NIH) Recommendations for Calcium Intake

Group/age (years)	Recommended calcium intake (mg)
Adolescents/young adults	
11–24	1200–1500
Women	
25–50	1000
Over 50 (postmenopausal)	
On estrogen	1000
Estrogen deficient	1500
Over 65	1500
Pregnant or nursing	1200–1500
Men	
25–65	1000
Over 65	1500

3. Moderation in caffeine intake
4. Moderation in salt (sodium) intake
5. Modification of the home environment to reduce the risk of falls

Cigarette smoke, alcohol, caffeine, and sodium are all associated with bone loss, to some degree (19–23). Modification of the home environment does not have to be extensive to reduce the risk of falls. Measures include removing throw rugs; eliminating electrical extension cords from walk areas; installing automatic night-lights in the bedroom, bath, and kitchen; and installing safety bars in the bath. Only the installation of safety bars in the bath requires any expertise or potential expense. The bars themselves are not expensive, but they must be installed into the studs of the wall with long screws in order to support the weight of the body. These are all relatively simple measures that can be life saving.

CALCIUM, VITAMIN D, AND EXERCISE

Nonprescription interventions that are appropriate for most, but not all, women are obtaining adequate calcium and vitamin D and regular weight-bearing or resistance exercise. There are several different sets of recommendations for calcium intake. The differences tend to be small and following any one of them is appropriate. Table 9-4 lists the recommendations for calcium intake from the 1994 National Institutes of Health (NIH)

Table 9-5
1997 National Academy of Science Recommendations for Calcium Intake

Group/age (yrs)	Recommended calcium intake (mg)
Adolescents/adults (both sexes)	
9–18	1300
19–50	1000
51+	1200
Pregnant or nursing women	
≤18	1300
19–50	1000

Consensus Conference on Calcium Intake (24). Table 9-5 lists the 1997 recommended intakes according to the National Academy of Science (25). The NOF has issued a blanket recommendation of 1200 mg/day for all adults (17).

Obtaining these recommended amounts of calcium from the diet alone is often difficult although it is the desirable means. Over-the-counter calcium supplements are an acceptable means of supplementing dietary calcium to ensure that the intake goals are met. Calcium supplements are relatively inexpensive. Most supplements are forms of calcium carbonate, but supplements of calcium citrate, calcium phosphate, and combinations of calcium lactate and gluconate are also available. All of these supplements with the exception of calcium citrate should be taken with food. Calcium citrate is best taken on an empty stomach. It is also important to note the milligrams of elemental calcium per tablet, because this is the important amount, not the milligrams of calcium salt. For example, a common strength of calcium carbonate tablet is 1250 mg of calcium carbonate. This tablet size provides 500 mg, not 1250 mg, of elemental calcium. Calcium-fortified foods and beverages are also useful in increasing dietary calcium intake. In addition to calcium-fortified bread, rice, and cereal, a variety of fruit juices are now fortified with calcium. Obtaining excessive amounts of calcium is not recommended. There is no proof that consuming amounts in excess of those recommended is beneficial. Furthermore, this may also increase the likelihood of developing a kidney stone if excessively large amounts of calcium are excreted into the urine.

Patients should always be asked if they have ever had a kidney stone or been told to avoid foods high in calcium before recommending an increase in dietary calcium or calcium supplements. Patients who have should be encouraged to discuss this issue with their physician before proceeding on their own.

Vitamin D is important for calcium absorption and metabolism, but it is not always necessary to consume a vitamin D supplement. It is certainly not necessary to have vitamin D and calcium in the same tablet. The 1997 National Academy of Science recommendations for vitamin D intake called for 200 International Units (I.U.) per day for both sexes from ages 14 to 50 and 400 I.U. for ages 51 to 70 (25). After age 70, 600 I.U. was recommended. Most over-the-counter multivitamin preparations contain 400 I.U. of vitamin D. Such a multivitamin is a reasonable choice for women age 51 and older to ensure adequate vitamin D intake. The vitamin D in such preparations must undergo chemical conversions in the liver and kidney before becoming biologically active. Because of this delay, any vitamin D combined with a calcium supplement does not actually affect the absorption of the calcium in that supplement; its actions will begin later.

Exercise is important in bone health. The most beneficial forms of exercise for the skeleton are weight-bearing exercise and resistance exercise. Weight-bearing exercise is any type of exercise that forces the skeleton to support the weight of the body. For example, walking is a weight-bearing exercise, whereas swimming is not. Resistance exercise is exercise in which the muscles push or pull against a resistance. Such resistance can be in the form of weight, tension, or air pressure. This is the type of exercise that is performed with the use of machines or free weights. There are restrictions on the type of exercise that women with osteoporosis should perform. High-impact exercises may place a fragile spine at risk for fracture and should be avoided. These include running, rope jumping, and high-impact aerobics. Any type of exercise in which the risk of falling is increased should be avoided. Exercises that require repeated or resisted trunk flexion should also be avoided because this may increase the risk of spine fracture.* Such exercises include traditional sit-ups and toe-touches. Trunk or spine extension exercises are both safe and recommended.

Prescription Interventions

The prescription medications used in osteoporosis are all antiresorptive medications. Some are approved by the FDA for the prevention of osteopo-

---

*Trunk flexion refers to bending forward from the waist with the back rounded.

Table 9-6
FDA-Approved Estrogen Preparations for Prevention of Osteoporosis

Premarin®	Estratest®
Prempro®	Estratest H.S®
Premphase®	Ortho-Est®
Ogen®	Climara®
Estrace®	Ortho-Prefest™
Estraderm™	femHRT®
Estratab®	Activella™

rosis, for the treatment of osteoporosis, or both. An antiresorptive agent is a medication that primarily inhibits bone loss rather than stimulates new bone formation. Increases in the measured bone density are observed with these agents, which may seem contradictory if the agents primarily inhibit bone loss. Part of this increase is attributed to the agent stopping additional bone loss while the skeleton rebuilds bone naturally. This rebuilding of bone is not directly stimulated by the antiresorptive agent. Agents that have been approved by the FDA for the prevention of bone loss or the prevention of osteoporosis have been shown to inhibit bone loss. Agents that are FDA approved for the treatment of osteoporosis have been shown in clinical trials to reduce the risk of fractures. Physicians are not restricted by these approvals from using a medication to treat osteoporosis that has been approved only for prevention and vice versa if it is deemed appropriate to do so.

ESTROGEN REPLACEMENT

An increasing number of estrogen replacement preparations are approved for the prevention of osteoporosis. The list has grown rapidly over the last few years and will undoubtedly continue to grow. The approval for the prevention of osteoporosis does not extend to every form of estrogen replacement available by prescription. It is given only to those preparations that have provided information from clinical trials to the FDA demonstrating that the particular preparation at a specific dose inhibits bone loss. Table 9-6 provides a list of approved preparations. Premarin® was previously approved for the treatment of osteoporosis as well. This approval was rescinded, not because the preparation was shown to be ineffective, but because there were inadequate data to prove its efficacy by current standards. Many physicians will appropriately use estrogen preparations in the treatment of osteoporosis as well as prevention.

THE SELECTIVE ESTROGEN RECEPTOR MODULATOR RALOXIFENE

Raloxifene, or Evista®, was approved for the prevention of osteoporosis in 1997 and the treatment of osteoporosis in 1999. The recommended dose is one 60-mg tablet by mouth once a day. In a very large clinical trial known as the MORE (Multiple Outcomes of Raloxifene Evaluation) study, women who received 60 mg of raloxifene/day for 3 years had a 2.1% increase in posteroanterior (PA) lumbar spine bone density and a 2.6% increase in femoral neck bone density compared with women who received a placebo *(26)*. Compared to their baseline bone density, women receiving 60 mg of raloxifene/day had an increase of approximately 3% at the PA lumbar spine and 1% at the femoral neck. Most important, there was a 30% reduction in the risk of new spine fractures in these women over the course of the 3-year study. Raloxifene does not stimulate the endometrium and cause menstrual bleeding. It also does not appear to have any beneficial effect on hot flashes and conveys a risk of thromboembolic events similar to estrogen *(27)*.

SYNTHETIC SALMON CALCITONIN

Synthetic salmon calcitonin in an injectable form has been available for the treatment of osteoporosis in the United States since 1984. In 1995, a nasal spray formulation was approved for the treatment of osteoporosis in women more than 5 years postmenopausal. Both the injectable form and nasal spray are available by prescription. The injectable synthetic salmon calcitonin is given in a dose of 100 I.U. subcutaneously daily. The recommended dose of the nasal spray is 200 I.U. once a day. One spray delivers the recommended dose. The results of the PROOF (Prevent Recurrence of Osteoporotic Fractures) trial, a 5-year clinical trial evaluating the efficacy of synthetic salmon calcitonin nasal spray, were published in 2000 *(28)*. The women who received 200 I.U. of synthetic salmon calcitonin nasal spray had small increases of slightly greater than 1% in PA lumbar spine bone density compared with their baseline value over the course of the 5-year trial. This increase was significantly different from the placebo group only at the end of years 1 and 2. Over the course of the 5-year study, however, the women receiving 200 I.U. of synthetic salmon calcitonin nasal spray had a 33% reduction in the risk of new spine fractures.

At present, Miacalcin® is the only brand of synthetic salmon calcitonin nasal spray available for prescription use in the United States. The medication is delivered by a pump-spray assembly. The vial should be kept refrigerated prior to first use, after which it can remain at room temperature. The medication can be used without regard to meals or time of day. There are no known drug interactions, and no adjustments are necessary based on age or kidney function.

BISPHOSPHONATES

Bisphosphonates are quite similar to pyrophosphate, a substance normally found in bone. The first bisphosphonate was etidronate (Didronel®). Although etidronate has never been approved for the prevention or treatment of osteoporosis, early research using etidronate to treat osteoporosis helped spur the development of more potent bisphosphonates for use in osteoporosis *(29,30)*. Two bisphosphonates are currently available by prescription for both the prevention and treatment of osteoporosis: alendronate (Fosamax®) and risedronate (Actonel™).

Alendronate is approved for the prevention and treatment of osteoporosis in women as well as for the treatment of osteoporosis in men. When used to treat osteoporosis, the recommended dose was originally one 10-mg tablet once a day. Recent data, however, have demonstrated that it is equally effective to give 70 mg only once a week *(31)*. Both the 10 mg daily and 70 mg once weekly doses are now approved for the treatment of osteoporosis in women and men. The recommended dose when used for the prevention of osteoporosis is one 5-mg tablet once a day or 35 mg once a week. The medication must be taken before breakfast, after an overnight fast. It must be taken with a full glass of water alone, and no other beverage, food, or medication should be consumed for at least 30 minutes. It is also important that the patient remain up after taking the medication and not go back to bed. These instructions are necessary to ensure that the medication is absorbed properly and that any chance of reflux into the esophagus, where it could cause irritation, is minimized. There are no known adverse drug interactions with alendronate, but it is not recommended for individuals with renal insufficiency.

The efficacy of alendronate is unquestioned. In the 3-year Fracture Intervention Trial (FIT), women receiving 10 mg of alendronate daily had a 47% reduction in their risk of having new spine fractures compared with women receiving a placebo *(32)*. There was also a 51% reduction in the risk of hip fractures. Bone density at the PA lumbar spine increased by more than 8% and at the femoral neck by approximately 3% compared with baseline in women receiving alendronate over the 3-year study period. The effects of 7 years of continuous treatment with alendronate have been published showing an average increase of 11.4% at the spine from baseline

(33). In another 3-year study, alendronate was shown to be effective in preventing bone loss in recently menopausal women with lumbar spine bone densities within 2 SDs of the young adult peak bone density *(34)*. In that study, alendronate given in a dose of 5 or 10 mg/day prevented bone loss from the spine and hip.

The effectiveness of adding alendronate to ongoing hormone replacement was investigated in a 2-year study known as the FACET (Fosamax Addition to Continiung Estrogen Therapy) study *(35)*. In women who received 10 mg of alendronate in addition to their ongoing hormone replacement, there was a 2.6% greater increase in PA spine BMD and a 2.7% greater increase in trochanteric BMD compared with women who simply continued hormone replacement. The combination appeared safe as well. This study was not designed to evaluate potential reductions in fracture risk from combination therapy.

Alendronate has been approved for the treatment of osteoporosis in men. In a 2-year study of 241 men with osteoporosis, alendronate at a dose of 10 mg/day resulted in significant increases in bone density at the spine and hip *(36)*. The average increase from baseline at the PA lumbar spine was 7.1% and at the femoral neck, 2.5%. The incidence of vertebral fracture was also reduced in the men receiving alendronate. Testosterone levels had no apparent influence on the effectiveness of alendronate.

Risedronate is also approved for the prevention and treatment of osteoporosis in women. A dose of 5 mg given once per day is recommended for either prevention or treatment. Like alendronate, risedronate should be given after an overnight fast, with only a full glass of water. Nothing other than water should be consumed for at least 30 minutes after taking risedronate, and the patient should remain up after taking it. No significant drug interactions are known to occur with risedronate, and no alterations in dose are necessary solely on the basis of age. Like alendronate, risedronate is not recommended in individuals with renal insufficiency.

The efficacy of risedronate in reducing spine fracture risk has been demonstrated in two large clinical trials, collectively called the VERT trials *(37,38)*. Both of these trials were 3-year studies involving several thousand women with preexisting spine fractures. In the US trial, women who received 5 mg of risedronate had a 41% reduction in their risk of new spine fracture *(37)*. Bone density increased at the lumbar spine by 5.2% and at the femoral neck by 1.6% compared with baseline over the 3-year study. In the multinational or European trial, women who received 5 mg of risedronate had a 49% reduction in the risk of new spine fractures *(38)*. Bone density at the spine increased by approximately 7% and at the femoral neck by approximately 2% from baseline by the end of the study.

Risedronate also prevents bone loss in recently menopausal women. In a 2-year study of women within 3 years of menopause, 5 mg of risedronate/day resulted in small but significant increases in lumbar spine and femoral neck bone density, whereas women receiving a placebo lost bone density at those sites *(39)*.

Both bisphosphonates must be taken only with water, because all bisphosphonates are very poorly absorbed when taken by mouth. It is imperative that nothing other than water be used when taking the tablet and that nothing other than water be consumed for at least 30 minutes. Any other beverage or food consumed during that time would potentially result in a failure to absorb an adequate amount of the medication. The stomach must be empty at the time the medication is taken, so that no previously consumed food, beverage, or medication is present to interfere with the absorption of the bisphosphonate. That is why the medication should be taken after an overnight fast and before breakfast.

The bisphosphonates have the potential to cause irritation of the esophagus. It is for this reason that patients are encouraged to consume a full glass of water to ensure passage of the tablet from the esophagus into the stomach. This is also why patients are advised to remain up after taking the medication, in order to reduce any risk of reflux of the medication into the esophagus. Because of the potential for esophageal irritation, oral bisphosphonates such as alendronate and risedronate are generally not recommended for use in individuals who have difficulty swallowing or preexisting esophageal disorders that might make passage of the tablet into the stomach more difficult. These are disorders such as delayed esophageal emptying, esophageal strictures, and esophageal ulceration.

Although these restrictions on the use of bisphosphonates are appropriately emphasized, note that both bisphosphonates are very safe overall. In all the major trials in which women taking either alendronate or risedronate were compared with women taking a placebo, no increase in gastrointestinal side effects has been demonstrated in women taking either bisphosphonate. Gastrointestinal complaints occur fairly frequently in such research trials as they do in the general population, but they are equally frequent in women not taking the bisphosphonate as in those who are *(32,37,38)*. This suggests that gastrointestinal complaints are common in the age group of women in whom these drugs are likely to be used; it does not suggest that the drugs are the cause. The bisphosphonates alendronate and risedronate are two of the most efficacious and well-studied drugs available for the prevention and treatment of osteoporosis. Their use should not be discontinued prematurely because of minor gastrointestinal complaints.

PATIENT EDUCATION MATERIALS

Densitometry facilities may wish to develop their own patient education materials in osteoporosis and densitometry, but many brochures and pamphlets are available at no cost from local pharmaceutical representatives. In some instances, these materials can be personalized for the densitometry facility. Such materials will also generally contain some mention of the particular product or medication manufactured by the company but these references are usually kept to a minimum. Publications suitable for patients are also available from the NOF.[†††] A variety of books on osteoporosis are available at local book stores. The third edition of *The Osteoporosis Handbook*, by Sydney Lou Bonnick, MD, is highly recommended.

REFERENCES

1. Consensus Development Conference. (1991) Prophylaxis and treatment of osteoporosis. *Am. J. Med.* **90**, 107–110.
2. Peck, W. A. (1993) Consensus development conference: diagnosis, prophylaxis, and treatment of osteoporosis. *Am. J. Med.* **94**, 646–650.
3. World Health Organization. (1994) Assessment of fracture risk and its application to screening for postmenopausal osteoporosis: report of a WHO study group. WHO Technical Report Series, WHO, Geneva.
4. Melton, L. J., Chrischilles, E. A., Cooper, C., Lane, A. W., Riggs, B. L. (1992) How many women have osteoporosis? *J. Bone Miner. Res.* **7**, 1005–1010.
5. Melton, L. J. (1995) How many women have osteoporosis now? *J. Bone Miner. Res.* **10**, 175–177.
6. Chrischilles, E. A., Butler, C. D., Davis, C. S., Wallace, R. B. (1991) A model of lifetime osteoporosis impact. *Arch. Intern. Med.* **151**, 2026–2032.
7. Ray, N. F., Chan, J. K., Thamer, M., Melton, L. J. (1997) Medical expenditures for the treatment of osteoporotic fractures in the United States: a report from the National Osteoporosis Foundation. *J. Bone Miner. Res.* **12**, 24–35.
8. Schlaich, C., Minne, H. W., Bruckner, T., et al. (1998) Reduced pulmonary function in patients with spinal osteoporotic fractures. *Osteoporos. Int.* **8**, 261–267.
9. Marotolli, R. A., Berkman, L. F., Cooney, L. M. (1992) Decline in physical function following hip fracture. *J. Am. Geriatr. Soc.* **40**, 861–866.
10. Cummings, S. R., Kelsey, J. L., Nevitt, M. C., O'Dowd, K. J. (1985) Epidemiology of osteoporosis and osteoporotic fractures. *Epidemiol. Rev.* **7**, 178–208.
11. Bonnick, S. L., Nichols, D. L., Sanborn, C. F., Lloyd, K., Payne, S. G., Lewis, L., Reed, C. A. (1997) Dissimilar spine and femoral *z*-scores in premenopausal women. *Calcif. Tissue Int.* **61**, 263–265.
12. Hansen, M. A. (1994) Assessment of age and risk factors on bone density and bone turnover in healthy premenopausal women. *Osteoporos. Int.* **4**, 123–128.

[†††]See Appendix I for contact information.

13. Rodin, A., Murby, B., Smith, M. A., et al. (1990) Premenopausal bone loss in the lumbar spine and neck of the femur: a study of 225 Caucasian women. *Bone* **11,** 1–5.
14. Lloyd, T. Martel, J. K., Rollings, N., et al. (1996) The effect of calcium supplementation and Tanner stage on bone density and area in teenage women. *Osteoporos. Int.* **6,** 276–283.
15. Slemenda, C. W., Miller, J. Z., Hui, S. L., Reister, T. K., Johnston, C. C. (1991) The role of physical activity in the development of skeletal mass in children. *J. Bone Miner. Res.* **6,** 1227–1233.
16. Melton, L. J. (1993) Epidemiology of age-related fractures, in *The Osteoporotic Syndrome* (Avioli, L.V., ed.), Wiley-Liss, New York, pp. 17–38.
17. National Osteoporosis Foundation. (1998) *Physician's Guide to Prevention and Treatment of Osteoporosis,* Excerpta Medica, Belle Mead, NJ.
18. Health Care Financing Administration, Department of Health and Human Services. (1998). Medicare program: Medicare coverage of and payment for bone mass measurements. *Fed. Reg.* 42 CFR, Part 410.
19. Kiel, D. P., Baron, J. A., Anderson, J. J., Hannan, M. T., Felson, D. T. (1992) Smoking eliminates the protective effect of oral estrogens on the risk for hip fracture among women. *Ann. Intern. Med.* **116,** 716–721.
20. Cornuz, J., Feskanich, D., Willett, W. C., Colditz, G. A. (1999) Smoking, smoking cessation and risk of hip fracture in women. *Am. J. Med.* **106,** 311–314.
21. Barger-Lux, J. J., Heaney, R. P., Stegman, M. R. (1990) Effects of moderate caffeine intake on the calcium economy of premenopausal women. *Am. J. Clin. Nutr.* **52,** 722–725.
22. Bikle, D. D., Genant, H. K., Cann, C., Recker, R. R., Halloran, B. P., Strewler, G. J. (1985) Bone disease in alcohol abuse. *Ann. Intern. Med.* **103,** 42–48.
23. Burger, H., Grobbee, D. E., Drucke, T. (2000) Osteoporosis and salt intake. *Nutr. Metab. Cardiovasc. Dis.* **10,** 46–53.
24. (1994) Optimal calcium intake. *N.I.H. Consens. Statement,* **vol. 12,** pp. 1–31.
25. Yates, A. A., Schlicker, S. A., Suitor, C. W. (1998) Dietary reference intakes: the new basis for recommendations for calcium and related nutrients, B vitamins, and choline. *J. Am. Diet. Assoc.* **98,** 699–706.
26. Ettinger, B., Black, D. M., Mitlak, B. H., et al. (1999) Reduction of vertebral fracture risk in postmenopausal women with osteoporosis treated with raloxifene. *JAMA* **282,** 637–645.
27. Delmas, P. D., Bjarnason, N. H., Mitlak, B. H., et al. (1997) Effect of raloxifene on bone mineral density, serum cholesterol concentrations, and uterine endometrium in postmenopausal women. *N. Engl. J. Med.* **337,** 1641–1647.
28. Chesnut, C. H., Silverman, S., Andriano, K., et al. (2000) A randomized trial of nasal spray salmon calcitonin in postmenopausal women with established osteoporosis: the prevent recurrence of osteoporotic fractures study. *Am. J. Med.* **109,** 267–276.
29. Watts, N. B., Harris, S. T., Genant, H. K., et al. (1990) Intermittent cyclical etidronate treatment of postmenopausal osteoporosis. *N. Engl. J. Med.* **323,** 73–79.
30. Storm, T., Thamsborg, G., Steiniche, T., Genant, H. K., Sørensen, O. H. (1990) Effect of intermittent cyclical etidronate therapy of bone mass and fracture rate in women with postmenopausal osteoporosis. *N. Engl. J. Med.* **322,** 1265–1271.
31. Schnitzer, T., Bone, H. G., Crepaldi, G., et al. (2000) Therapeutic equivalence of alendronate 70 mg once-weekly and alendronate 10 mg daily in the treatment of osteoporosis. *Aging Clin. Exp. Res.* **12,** 1–12.
32. Black, D. M., Cummings, S. R., Karpf, D. B., et al. (1996) Randomised trial of

effect of alendronate on risk of fracture in women with existing fractures. *Lancet* **348**, 1535–1541.

33. Tonino, R. P., Meunier, P. J., Emkey, R., et al. (2000) Skeletal benefits of alendronate: 7-year treatment of postmenopausal osteoporotic women. Phase III osteoporosis treatment study group. *J. Clin. Endocrinol. Metab.* **85**, 3109–3115.

34. McClung, M., Clemmesen, B., Daifotis, A., et al. (1998) Alendronate prevents postmenopausal bone loss in women without osteoporosis. *Ann. Intern. Med.* **128**, 253–261.

35. Lindsay, R., Cosman, F., Lobo, F. A., et al. (1999) Addition of alendronate to ongoing hormone replacement therapy in the treatment of osteoporosis: a randomized, controlled clinical trial. *J. Clin. Endocrinol. Metab.* **84**, 3076–3081.

36. Orwoll, E., Ettinger, M., Weiss, S., et al. (2000) Alendronate for the treatment of osteoporosis in men. *N. Engl. J. Med.* **343**, 604–610.

37. Harris, S. T., Watts, N. B., Genant, H. K., et al. (1999) Effects of risedronate treatment on vertebral and nonvertebral fractures in women with postmenopausal osteoporosis. *JAMA* **282**, 1344–1352.

38. Reginster, J.Y., Minne, H.W., Sorensen, O.H., et al. (2000) Randomized trial of the effects of risedronate on vertebral fractures in women with established postmenopausal osteoporosis. *Osteoporos. Int.* **11**, 83–91.

39. Hooper, M., Ebeling, P., Roberts, A., et al. (1999) Risedronate prevents bone loss in early postmenopausal women. *Calcif. Tissue Int.* **64** (Abstract P-80), S69.

10 Interpretation of Bone Densitometry Data

CONTENTS

The physician is always ultimately responsible for the interpretation of bone densitometry data. The ability of technologists to perform their duties, however, is only enhanced by understanding what the physician will attempt to do with the data that they provide. The circumstances in which bone densitometry is often performed are also quite different from those in which other diagnostic procedures are usually performed. Unlike having a chest X ray, in which the procedure is over in a few seconds, the patient is often asked to sit or lie down for several minutes during a bone density study. The technologist is not physically separated from the patient by a protective barrier but usually seated only a few feet away. It is inevitable that the patient will ask questions about the test and the nature of the results. The technologist should be able to respond to these questions appropriately while ultimately deferring to the diagnostic judgment of the physician. It is also true that occasionally the technologist must make decisions independently regarding the choice of skeletal site to measure, the technical acceptability of the study, and the timing of return visits. An understanding of how the data are to be used is crucial to making these decisions.

THE RESULTS

The type of information obtained from the various bone densitometry devices may appear different, but the nature of the information is the same. With only a few exceptions, the information can be categorized as follows:

- The skeletal image.
- The measured and calculated bone density parameters.
- Comparisons to the reference database.
  —% Comparisons.
  —Standard score comparisons.
- Standardized bone mineral density (sBMD).
- Age-regression graph.
- Assignment of diagnostic category based on World Health Organization (WHO) criteria.

The exact location of this information on the computer screen or on the printout varies from device to device, but the nature of the information does not.

The Skeletal Image

All of today's X-ray densitometers provide an image of the region of the skeleton being studied. Some, but not all, ultrasound densitometers do so as well. These images should always be closely examined for the possible presence of artifacts that would affect the accuracy of the study and the interpretation of the data. If problems are suspected from a review of the image, it is appropriate for the technologist to contact the physician to ask whether another site should be studied. At the very least, it is appropriate for the technologist to flag the study in some way, to alert the physician to possible problems. Most of the skeletal images created during a bone densitometry study are not approved by the Food and Drug Administration (FDA) for use in making structural diagnoses. Plain films are required if it is necessary to confirm the suspected skeletal abnormalities. Nevertheless, it is important that the images be reviewed for possible structural problems. This situation occurs most often with studies of the posteroanterior (PA) lumbar spine.

As noted in Chapter 3, the presence of osteophytes, facet sclerosis, or compression fractures will increase the measured BMD. While the device is accurately measuring the amount of mineral in the beam path such that the measurement cannot truly be said to be inaccurate, clearly the interpretation of the bone density data in the context of osteoporosis will be affected. The precision of future measurements at that site will also be poorer. As a consequence, if the technologist is aware that the study is being done to establish a baseline value for future measurements, it would be appropriate to contact the physician to explain the potential problem to ask whether another skeletal site should be measured.

The presence of a suspected fracture has additional significance in assigning the patient's diagnosis and the interpretation of risk for future fracture. In a postmenopausal Caucasian woman, the presence of a fracture combined with a bone density that is 2.5 standard deviations (SDs) or more below the average peak bone density of the young adult will result in a diagnosis of severe osteoporosis rather than just osteoporosis. In addition, many studies have shown that the risk for future fracture is greater than that implied by the bone density alone once a fracture has occurred (1–4). For example, the PA lumbar spine image from the dual-energy X-ray absorptiometry (DXA) study shown in Fig. 10-1 clearly suggests the presence of a compression fracture at L3. A review of the individual BMD values for each vertebra also clearly shows a dramatic increase in the BMD between L2 and L3 that is much greater than expected. The presence of a fracture at L3 should be confirmed with plain X rays because this image is not FDA approved for use in making structural diagnoses. Nevertheless, suspicion should be aroused by these findings. The increase in BMD at L3 will increase the L2–L4 BMD on which comparisons to the reference database will be made. The higher T-score could result in an incorrect diagnosis. It is quite likely that this patient is actually osteoporotic rather than osteopenic, as the T-score in Fig. 10-1 suggests. The presence of a fracture also implies that the patient is at much greater risk of future fracture than the bone density alone implies. It would be entirely appropriate for the technologist to note that there appears to be a structural problem at L3 and that the BMD at L3 is unusually high compared with L2 and L4. Without going any further, the technologist would be able to alert the physician to potential problems in the interpretation of the data.

Structural diagnoses can be made using the new IVA™ application from Hologic and the LVA™ application from GE Lunar, in which the

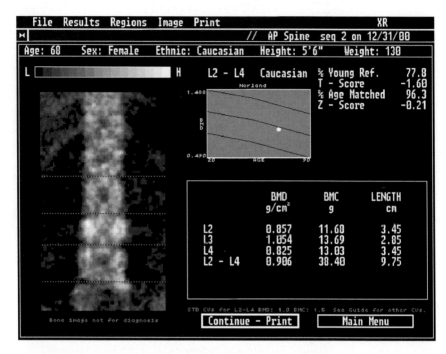

Fig. 10-1. Norland XR-series PA lumbar spine study. A review of the skeletal image suggests a loss of height and increased density at L3. The values for the individual vertebrae also suggest a much greater increase in density between L2 and L3 than normal. These findings are suggestive of fracture at L3 although plain films would be required to prove this. The L2–L4 BMD will be increased by the process at L3.

entire spine is imaged. These applications are available only on specific models from the respective manufacturers. If these applications are available and a structural abnormality in the spine is suspected, the physician can be contacted for permission to proceed with spine imaging to confirm the presence and nature of the suspected abnormality. Figure 10-2 is an IVA™ image from the Hologic Delphi™ that shows a wedge fracture at L1.

Measured and Calculated Bone Density Parameters

The measured and calculated parameters for the regions of interest (ROIs) are displayed on the computer screen at the conclusion of the analysis phase of the bone density study. Remember that BMD is actually calculated from the measurements of bone mineral content (BMC) and area or volume, as described in Chapter 1. When multiple ROIs have been measured during a single study, the technologist must decide which

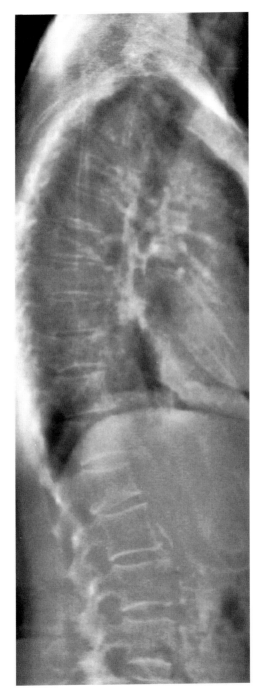

Fig. 10-2. Delphi IVA™ image of the lateral spine. The remarkable clarity of this image allows structural diagnoses to be made. A compression fracture is seen at L1 as well as aortic calcification anterior to the lower lumbar spine. This is a single energy X-ray image. (Photo courtesy of Hologic, Bedford, MA.)

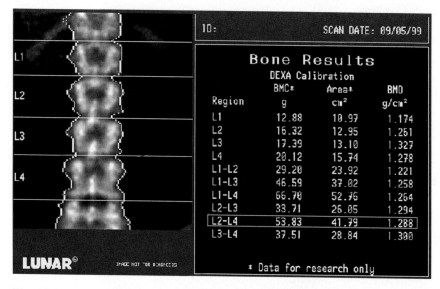

Table content:

Region	BMC* g	Area* cm²	BMD g/cm²
L1	12.88	10.97	1.174
L2	16.32	12.95	1.261
L3	17.39	13.10	1.327
L4	20.12	15.74	1.278
L1–L2	29.20	23.92	1.221
L1–L3	46.59	37.02	1.258
L1–L4	66.70	52.76	1.264
L2–L3	33.71	26.05	1.294
L2–L4	53.83	41.79	1.288
L3–L4	37.51	28.84	1.300

Fig. 10-3. PA lumbar spine GE Lunar DPX™ study. The measured parameters of BMC and area are shown for each individual vertebra and every possible combination of contiguous vertebrae. The BMD that is calculated by dividing the BMC by the area is also shown for each individual vertebra and every combination of contiguous vertebrae. The technologist can choose to emphasize any value, but the L1–L4 or L2–L4 BMD is preferred for reasons of statistical accuracy and precision.

region's parameters to emphasize. The calculated parameter for the region that is chosen will be highlighted and plotted on an age-regression graph. It is this value that will likely receive the physician's attention. As a consequence, it is imperative that the technologist select the correct region and the correct parameter for that region.

Figure 10-3 gives the measured and calculated values for each vertebra at the PA spine. Also shown are the values for each combination of contiguous vertebrae. On most devices, a "default" ROI is programmed into the software. This is the ROI that will be emphasized unless changed by the technologist. On the study shown in Fig. 10-3, the L2–L4 BMD is highlighted by default. If unchanged by the technologist, this value will be plotted on the age-regression graph and displayed prominently on the printout. For PA spine studies, it is preferable to use the BMD calculated from the measurement of three or four contiguous vertebrae as long as none of those vertebrae are affected by artifacts. The reason for selecting the three- or four-vertebral BMD over the BMD for only one or two vertebrae is that the accuracy and precision of the measurement are superior. The default ROI on central GE Lunar and Norland DXA devices at the spine is the L2–L4 BMD and on Hologic central DXA devices is L1–L4. If one of the vertebrae in these default regions is suspected of being structurally abnormal, it should be excluded from the calculation or the average from another set of contiguous vertebrae chosen. The preferable approach will depend on the type of densitometry device.

In the proximal femur, five different ROIs can be measured: the total hip (or total femur), femoral neck, Ward's area, trochanter, and shaft. The total hip ROI combines the femoral neck, Ward's area, trochanter, and shaft into one measurement. Because the combined area of all these regions that contribute to the total hip measurement is greater than the area of any one of these regions alone, the precision of the total hip measurement tends to be the best of any of the five regions. For this reason, many authorities prefer to emphasize the total hip ROI over the other regions in the proximal femur. This enthusiasm must be tempered by the recognition that any anticipated rate of change in the total hip ROI will tend to be slower than in the femoral neck. The combination of precision and rate of change, not precision alone, determines a site's utility for serial measurements.* Excellent precision can be obtained at the femoral neck at which greater rates of change are generally seen. Both regions are similarly useful in the prediction of fracture risk (5). As a consequence, we prefer to emphasize the femoral neck over the total hip. The technologist should consult with the supervising physician to determine which ROI is preferred. Ward's area is virtually never emphasized, because it is not used for diagnosis, fracture risk assessment, or monitoring of bone density. In research studies, Ward's area is a good predictor of fracture risk. Nevertheless, its utility in an individual is quite limited. The area defined by the densitometry computer software as constituting Ward's area is so small that the accuracy and precision of the measurement are extremely poor compared to the total hip and femoral neck.

At the forearm, many densitometers measure several different skeletal sites. It is also possible to obtain a measurement at one site of either the radius or ulna, or of both bones combined. The combined measurement, again because of the larger area being measured, generally offers better accuracy and precision than the single bone measurement. This makes the combined bone measurement preferable. The preferred site on either

---

*See Chapter 6 for a discussion of the interaction between precision and rate of change.

bone or both bones combined is highly dependent on the reason the measurement is being made. The more distal regions in the forearm such as the ultradistal, 8-mm, 10%, and distal ROIs are generally preferred for the diagnosis of osteoporosis.[†] If a patient is being evaluated for hyperparathyroidism, the proximal, one third, or 33% sites are preferred. The choice of site is influenced by the percentage of trabecular and cortical bone found at those sites. In diseases such as osteoporosis, in which trabecular bone loss is an early feature, the more trabecular distal sites are preferred. Hyperparathyroidism tends to have a pronounced effect on cortical bone, making the highly cortical proximal sites the better sites to measure in the forearm. If the patient has had a distal radial fracture or Colles' fracture, the BMD at the distal site may be increased by as much as 20% whereas the proximal site tends to be unaffected (6). In this circumstance, if for some reason the opposite arm cannot be measured, the proximal site is the site that more accurately reflects the patient's bone mineral status. For the prediction of fracture risk, any of the distal or proximal sites can be used. None of the forearm sites are generally used for monitoring therapy. This is not because of either poor accuracy or poor precision at any of the sites; rather, it is because the rate of change at the forearm sites tends to be so slow that the time needed before the least significant change (LSC) will have occurred is much too long to be clinically useful.[*]

Measurements of bone density at the calcaneus, phalanges, and metacarpals do not present the technologist with a variety of ROIs from which to choose. These are normally predetermined by the computer software. Total body bone density studies can be subdivided into all the various regions of the skeleton. The accuracy and precision of the total body bone density measurement are excellent. When the skeleton is divided into smaller regions (smaller within the context of the total body measurement) such as the lumbar spine or legs, the accuracy and precision of the measurement suffer. As a result, it is not recommended that the various regions of the skeleton from a total body bone density measurement be used for diagnosis or monitoring of therapy. The total body bone density measurement itself is, as noted in Chapter 3, a measure of predominantly cortical bone. As such, it is not particularly useful in the diagnosis of diseases that affect the more trabecular areas of the skeleton or in monitor-

---

[†]See Chapter 3 for a discussion of naming conventions for forearm bone density sites.

[‡]See Chapter 6 for a discussion of LSC.

ing changes in trabecular bone from the therapeutic agents used in the treatment of osteoporosis.

Comparisons to the Reference Database

The percentage comparisons and standard score comparisons were discussed in Chapter 1. The ROI that is selected by the technologist to be emphasized on the printout also determines which set of comparisons will be emphasized as well. The percentage comparisons and standard score comparisons are different expressions of the same thing. The % young adult comparison and the T-score both compare the patient's BMD with the peak BMD value that is expected for healthy young adults of the same sex. The % age-matched comparison and the z-score both compare the patient's BMD with the BMD that is expected for an individual of the same age and sex. One comparison is simply in the form of a percentage whereas the other indicates the number of SDs above or below the reference value. In clinical practice, the standard score comparisons have been given more importance than the percentage comparisons in diagnosis and prediction of fracture risk. This is largely the result of the application of the WHO criteria for diagnosing osteoporosis, which are based on the number of SDs from the average peak bone density of the young adult. These criteria are readily converted to T-scores, as shown in Appendix II. In addition, most of the data from fracture trials demonstrating the utility of bone mass measurements in predicting fracture risk are expressed as the increase in risk per SD decline in bone density. Once again, these data are easily used in conjunction with the T- or z-score.

It is just as important to avoid misinterpreting the percentage comparisons and standard scores as it is to interpret them correctly. The % young adult comparison and T-score should never be interpreted as indicating a certain magnitude of bone loss. For example, although a patient may be found to have a bone density that is 15% below the average peak BMD for a young adult, a 15% bone loss could be proven only if it was known that the patient's peak BMD was in fact identical to the average peak BMD to which the patient is being compared. It is, after all, quite possible that the patient developed a lower-than-average peak BMD and that the patient has lost no bone density at all. On the other hand, if the patient had developed a better-than-average peak bone density as a young adult, he or she might have actually experienced an even greater loss than 15%. It is simply not possible to come to any conclusion in this regard from a single bone mass measurement. The % age-matched comparison and the z-score can also be misinterpreted. Patients often ask how they compare to others their same age. This question generally follows being told that their % young-adult comparison or T-score is relatively poor. It is possible to have a favorable age-matched comparison or z-score while having a poor % young adult comparison or T-score, because bone loss tends to occur with advancing age. The fact that lower levels of bone density are expected at older ages should not be misconstrued as indicating the absence of a problem. This loss of bone is not desirable and certainly not beneficial. A good % age-matched comparison and good z-score can provide a false sense of security in the presence of the more important low young adult comparisons.

These comparisons to the reference database should never be used in serial bone mass measurements to determine whether a change has occurred in the patient's bone density. When a patient is being followed over time to determine whether bone loss is occurring or whether a therapy has caused an increase in bone density, it is the actual BMD values that should be compared from study to study. As discussed in Chapter 6, the significance of the change in the BMD is determined by the precision of the measurement and the desired level of statistical confidence.

The T-score is readily used to determine the WHO diagnostic category if the patient is a postmenopausal Caucasian woman. If the patient is a healthy premenopausal Caucasian woman, the WHO criteria should not be applied. This is because, in an otherwise healthy woman, a low bone mass may not indicate bone loss. It may only indicate a lower than average peak bone density that is being maintained. Although there may be less mass in her bones, it is highly unlikely that there is anything wrong with the architecture of the bones. The 1991 and 1993 Consensus Conference definitions of osteoporosis require microarchitectural deterioration of bone tissue in addition to low bone mass.[§] Microarchitectural deterioration is presumed in older women with low bone mass, but it should not be presumed in otherwise healthy younger women. Labeling such a woman as having a disease is inappropriate. It is useful to make her aware that her bone mass is lower than average so that she will take all the necessary steps to prevent bone loss in the future. In the absence of other criteria, the WHO criteria for postmenopausal Caucasian women are used in conjunction with bone density measurements in postmenopausal African American, Hispanic, and Asian women, although it is not entirely clear

---

[§]See Chapter 9 for a discussion of the 1991 and 1993 Consensus Conference definitions of osteoporosis.

if this is appropriate. Similarly, the criteria are also being used in mature Caucasian men. The z-score is not used for diagnostic purposes.

In predicting fracture risk, the guiding principle is that the risk of fracture approximately doubles for each SD decline in bone density *(7)*. This is generally true for any type of fracture or all fractures as measured at any skeletal site. Therefore, since the T-score indicates how many SDs below the average peak BMD the patient's bone density actually lies, it can be used to predict fracture risk. This is an exponential relationship. For example, if the T-score is −3, and the risk of fracture doubles for each SD decline in bone density, the patient's risk of fracture is increased eight-fold ($2 \times 2 \times 2$) compared with the individual who still has the bone density of a young adult. If the z-score is −2, the patient's risk of fracture is increased four-fold (2×2) compared with an individual of the same age. Neither of these approaches is ideal. Using the T-score in this fashion probably overestimates the patient's actual fracture risk. Using the z-score almost certainly underestimates the patient's fracture risk. The use of the T-score is common, but better ways of expressing fracture risk are actively being pursued.

Predictions of fracture risk that refer to the risk of having any type of osteoporotic fracture are called *global fracture risk predictions.* Predictions of the risk of having a specific type of fracture are called *site-specific fracture risk predictions.* For example, the prediction of the risk of spine fracture is a site-specific fracture risk prediction. Similarly, the prediction of the risk of hip fracture is a site-specific fracture risk prediction. Site-specific fracture risk predictions do not have to be based on the measurement of BMD at the potential fracture site. For example, a site-specific spine fracture risk assessment can be made based on the measurement of BMD at the femoral neck as well as at the spine. A doubling of fracture risk for each SD decline in bone density is used for global fracture prediction almost irrespective of where the measurement is being made. For site-specific fracture predictions, the increase in fracture risk per SD decline in bone density that is used does depend on where the measurement is being made. For the prediction of hip fracture, the increase in risk is 2.6-fold for each SD decline in bone density at the femoral neck and 2.7-fold at the total hip *(5)*. If the measurement is made at the heel, the increase in risk is 2-fold and at the distal radius, 2.6-fold *(8)*. For the prediction of spine fracture, the increase in risk is 1.9-fold for each SD decline in PA spine bone density *(8)*. If the measurement is made at the femoral neck, the increase in risk is 1.8-fold and at the midradius, 2.2-fold. The available information on the increase in fracture risk per SD decline in bone density comes from studies in women age 60 or older. It is not known if such information is directly applicable to younger, postmenopausal women or, certainly, younger premenopausal women. For this reason, assessments of fracture risk based on bone mass measurements are most appropriately made in women age 60 and older.

Standardized BMD

The sBMD, reported in milligrams/square centimeter, is available as an option for the DXA L2–L4 PA spine BMD and the total hip BMD. The technologist can usually activate or deactivate this option by adjusting the settings of the software. As noted in Chapter 1, it was hoped that the sBMD would make possible direct comparisons of spine and proximal femur BMDs that were obtained on central devices from different manufacturers. The sBMD is not used for diagnosis, fracture risk assessment, or serial monitoring. In using the sBMD to compare values from two different machines, both machine's native BMD values should be converted to the sBMD value. The two sBMD values can then be compared. Because there is a margin of error in these conversions, at least a 3% difference in the sBMD values should be anticipated even when the bone density has not changed between the two measurements. This margin of error makes the sBMD difficult to use clinically because the conclusions that are drawn from such comparisons remain uncertain. One can only say that "there doesn't appear to have been any change" or that "this difference is larger than expected." More precise conclusions cannot be reached on the basis of the sBMD. The equations for the conversion of the manufacturer's PA spine and total hip BMD values to the sBMD are listed in Appendix VII.

Age-Regression Graph

The age-regression graph found on the printouts for all the different devices actually provides no additional information that cannot be obtained from the actual BMD and standard score comparisons. Patients often ask for an explanation of these colorful graphs, and, therefore, the technologist should be able to provide some insight into their meaning. Some recent additions to these graphs are also easily misinterpreted.

The horizontal axis of the age-regression graph reflects advancing age. The vertical axis indicates BMD in the units of the measurement. On some graphs, the vertical axis on the right indicates the T-score. The BMD of the default ROI or the ROI that has been selected by the technologist is

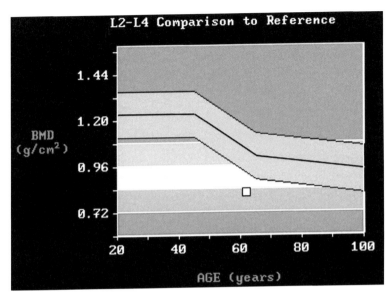

Fig. 10-4. Age-regression graph. The age-regression line is linear and flanked on either side by limits indicating change in bone density of ±1 SD from the age-matched predicted value. The patient's BMD is plotted above her age. From the graph, the patient appears to be approximately 62 years of age with a BMD slightly less than 0.84 g/cm². The T-score is poorer than −3 while the z-score is approximately−2.

plotted on the graph above the patient's age. A line indicates the expected value of BMD of the selected ROI for the age range represented on the graph. On some devices, depending on the skeletal site, this line tends to be flat in young adulthood and then drop sharply after the age of 45 or 50. On other devices, the line is more curvilinear. This line is called the *regression of bone density on age* or the *age regression*. The highest point on this line represents the peak bone density of the young adult. On some graphs, two other lines parallel the age-regression line on either side. These lines denote a change of either 1 or 2 SDs from the predicted value for any given age. The operator's manual must be consulted to determine whether a change of 1 or 2 SDs is being indicated. The patient's bone density can be visually compared with the peak bone density and the value that is predicted for their age. However, the actual bone density and the T- and z-scores could just as easily be read from the printout. Examples of age-regression graphs with linear or curvilinear age-regression lines are shown in Figs. 10-4 and 10-5.

On some of the newer versions of software, the background of these graphs is divided into areas that are colored red, yellow, and green, as

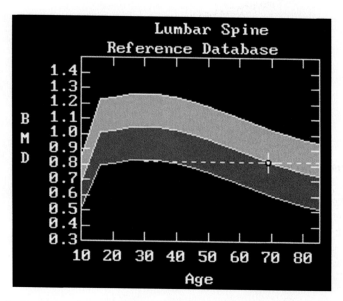

Fig. 10-5. Age-regression graph for a PA lumbar spine study. The age-regression line is curvilinear and flanked by limits indicating a change of ±2 SDs from the age-matched predicted value. The highest point on the age-regression appears to occur at approximately age 30, suggesting that that is the age of attainment of peak bone density at this site. The patient appears to be approximately 70 years of age with a BMD of 0.8 g/cm^2. The T-score is approximately −2 while the z-score is 0.

shown in Fig. 10-6. The dividing line between green and yellow is at a T-score of −1, and the dividing line between yellow and red is at a T-score of −2.5. These T-score cut points are intended to represent the dividing lines among the WHO categories of normal, osteopenia, and osteoporosis. This allows the technologist and physician to know immediately which WHO diagnostic category applies based on the measured bone density. Although possibly helpful, this can also be inappropriate. Notice on the generic graph in Fig. 10-6 that the divisions denoting the various diagnostic categories extend across the entire age range of the graph even though the WHO criteria are not intended for premenopausal women. Such graphs may also be seen in conjunction with bone density studies on men for whom the WHO criteria were not originally intended. An inappropriate diagnosis assigned by the computer can cause undue mental distress for the patient if not recognized and explained by the technologist or physician. Fracture risk assessments, based on the WHO diagnostic categories, also appear on age-regression graphs. Instead of the diagnostic categories of normal, osteopenia, and osteoporosis, risk

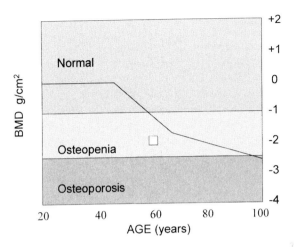

Fig. 10-6. Generic age-regression graph in which the background has been divided into three sections based on the T-score values of −1 and −2.5. This makes possible the assignment of the patient's BMD value to a WHO diagnostic category depending on where the BMD is plotted on the graph. While appropriate for postmenopausal Caucasian women, this may not be appropriate for others.

assessments of low, medium, and high appear in the green, yellow, and red areas that are again created by using the T-score cut points of −1 and −2.5. Unfortunately, like the WHO diagnostic category assignments, these colored areas representing levels of fracture risk extend across the entire age range represented on the graph. There are no data to support such an approach to the characterization of fracture risk in younger individuals. Consequently, this aspect of the age-regression graph must be interpreted with extreme caution.

Assignment of Diagnostic Category Based on WHO Criteria

As already noted, the assignment of diagnostic category has been incorporated into the age-regression graph on many bone densitometry devices. This can also be presented in a tabular form, as shown in Fig. 10-7. The diagnostic assignment on any computer printout should not be accepted automatically. It must be considered in light of the patient's age, sex, and race; the presence or absence of fractures; and the potential presence of confounding factors that might increase or decrease the measured BMD. Considerations of age, sex, and race have been previously discussed. If it is known that a fracture exists and the bone density is 2.5 SDs or more below the average peak bone density, the patient's diagnostic category

MetriScan Bone Mineral Density Report

Software Version 1.19

Exam Date	19/10/00 09:47 AM	Patient ID	01
Calibration Date	19/10/00 09:43 AM	Gender	Female
Instrument Serial #	100181	Age	50 years
Operator ID	1	Ethnic Group	Caucasian
Physician	_____	Patient Name	_____

Comments:

Image not for diagnosis

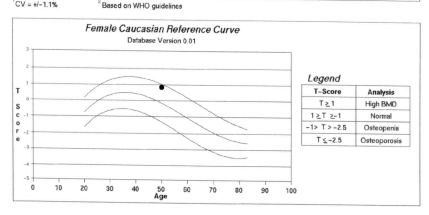

```
         60.46              66.07              53.61
        BMD results for individual fingers
```

BMD Test Results

	Estimated Relative BMD [1] (arbitrary units)	T-score (normative data)	Z-score (peer-matched data)
Result	60.04	0.75	0.84
Analysis	Normal [2]	105%	107%

[1] CV = +/-1.1%   [2] Based on WHO guidelines

Female Caucasian Reference Curve

Database Version 0.01

(T-score plotted against Age, curvilinear reference curve with patient point plotted near age 50, T-score ~1)

Legend

T-Score	Analysis
T ≥ 1	High BMD
1 ≥ T ≥ -1	Normal
-1 > T > -2.5	Osteopenia
T ≤ -2.5	Osteoporosis

Fig. 10-7. Alara MetriScan™ bone density report of a radiographic absorptiometry (RA) study of the phalanges. The middle phalanges of the index, long, and ring fingers are analyzed. The aluminum wedge is seen between the index and long fingers. The BMD is reported in arbitrary RA units along with the percentage comparisons and standard scores. A diagnostic assignment is made based on the T-score using WHO criteria. The curvilinear age-regression graph is seen, on which the patient's BMD is plotted above her age. Since the patient's z-score is given as 0.84, it is reasonable to assume that the limits surrounding the age-regression line represent a change in BMD of ±1 SD.

should change from osteoporosis to severe osteoporosis. On PA lumbar spine studies, suspected osteophytes, facet sclerosis, or other degenerative processes may increase the measured bone density, resulting in the assignment of a better diagnostic category than is justified (9). There is no substitute for clinical judgment when it comes to conveying what these numbers really mean. This does not mean that the measured and calculated parameters from these devices are not accurate or precise—they are. The medical implications of these numbers, however, must always be placed in the context of the individual patient.

CONFLICTING DIAGNOSES FROM MEASUREMENT OF MULTIPLE SITES

If a patient undergoes bone density testing of multiple skeletal sites or even of the same site by different techniques, it is quite likely that the various T-scores from the different tests will result in different diagnoses when the WHO criteria are used. For example, a postmenopausal Caucasian woman may undergo a DXA study of the PA lumbar spine and the proximal femur and be found to have a T-score at the PA lumbar spine of −1.5 and −2.6 at the femoral neck. By looking at each site individually and applying the WHO criteria, a diagnosis of osteopenia is appropriate at the spine while a diagnosis of osteoporosis is appropriate at the femoral neck. Another woman may have a DXA bone density measurement of her forearm and be found to have a T-score at the 33% combined forearm site of −0.9. A day later she may have an ultrasound study of the calcaneus at which time the T-score is found to be −2.0. A DXA study of the proximal femur in this same woman is −2.8. Depending on the site and technique, this woman could be classified as normal, osteopenic, or osteoporotic.

The recognition of this dilemma is not new. The WHO observed in 1994 that individuals would be classified differently depending on the site measured and the technique employed to make the measurement (10). This situation is created by three basic problems. First, the various skeletal sites need not do exactly the same thing at the same time. They may, in fact, be quite different from one another because of differences in weight bearing or differences in the percentages of cortical and trabecular bone. Some disease processes may preferentially affect one type of bone over the other. Second, different techniques may actually measure biologically different quantities. For example, the three-dimensional measurement of the spine made with quantitative computed tomography (QCT) can isolate trabecular from cortical bone. The two-dimensional spine measurement made with DXA cannot. The QCT measurement, then, is 100% trabecular bone whereas the DXA measurement may contain only 66% trabecular bone. The measurement of speed of sound or broadband ultrasound attenuation (BUA) with ultrasound may be biologically quite different from the measurement of bone mass with DXA. Third, there are differences in the reference databases that are the basis for the calculation of the percentage comparisons and the standard scores. Remember that the T-score reflects the number of SDs above or below the average peak bone density of the young adult that the patient's bone density lies. The T-score is, therefore, dependent on two quantities derived from the reference database: the value for the average peak bone density of the young adult and the value for the SD. The calculation of the SD itself is, in part, dependent on the number of individuals who were studied to create the reference database. In creating the reference databases for all the various bone density devices, each manufacturer has, of necessity, used a different population of individuals for each skeletal site. The criteria for participation in the reference population could vary from manufacturer to manufacturer, as could the number of individuals who were included. And, finally, once the studies were completed, different statistical methods may have been used to ultimately create the reference databases. When all three of these issues are considered, it is not surprising that different T-scores are encountered when measurements are made at multiple skeletal sites.

Differences in the percentage comparisons at the proximal femur among central devices were noted in the medical literature as early as 1992 *(11,12)*. Concern was raised in 1996 about the differences in T-scores and diagnostic assignments based on those T-scores at the proximal femur when different devices were used *(13)*. This led to the incorporation of the National Health and Nutrition Examination Survey (NHANES) III femur database by the manufacturers of central devices, as discussed in Chapter 1. With this common database, and therefore the same peak BMD and SD on which to base the calculation of the T-score, the diagnostic discrepancies were minimized.

The diagnostic discrepancies among other sites when measured by the same type of device from different manufacturers or by different techniques still remain a clinical problem. In a study using one central DXA device and the manufacturer-supplied databases, the percentage of women diagnosed as osteoporotic varied from 19.3 to 75%, depending on which skeletal site was used to make the diagnosis *(14)*. In another study in which only one central device was used but a common database for all sites was created by the researchers, the percentages of women diagnosed as osteoporotic still varied widely from 11 to 45.7%, depending on which site was measured *(15)*. In a similar study that included ultrasound measurements of the calcaneus as well as DXA measurements of other regions of the skeleton, significant differences in the percentages of women diagnosed as osteoporotic again resulted, depending on the site and technique used *(16)*.

Efforts are under way by a joint committee of the National Osteoporosis Foundation and the International Society for Clinical Densitometry to create a "T-score equivalent" to reduce the clinical confusion caused by discrepant T-scores. It is hoped that tables will be created to allow the technologist and physician to look at a table of T-scores for a specific device and site and determine what the "equivalent" T-score at the hip or spine would be. The equivalence would be based on the T-score at the hip or spine that implies the same level of risk for fracture as the T-score at the site that was actually measured. For example, an ultrasound study of the calcaneus might result in a T-score of −2 based on the BUA measurement. This would be equivalent to a DXA T-score of −2.5 at the femoral neck because both T-scores are associated with the same risk of hip fracture.* The development of T-score equivalents is eagerly awaited by the densitometry community.

REPORT REVIEW

A review of several different types of densitometry printouts will illustrate the similarities in the type of information provided on each report and also provide an opportunity to review some of the attributes of the various skeletal sites and techniques.

Figure 10-7 is a report from an Alara Metriscan™ study of the phalanges. This peripheral device employs RA and measures the middle phalanges of the index, long, and ring fingers. The radiation exposure to the patient is less than 0.001 μSv according to the manufacturer.‡ The phalanges themselves can be characterized as being part of the appendicular, peripheral, non-weight-bearing skeleton and predominantly cortical in composition. The skeletal image of the phalanges can be seen as well as

---

*These numbers are used only for the purpose of this example and should not be used clinically at this time.

‡See Chapter 4 for manufacturer descriptions of the various technologies.

the aluminum wedge that is used for comparison. The BMD in arbitrary RA units is reported as 60.04. Standard score and percentage comparisons are also given as well as the WHO diagnostic classification that is based on the reported T-score. The WHO criteria are given in tabular form in the lower right-hand corner of the report. The age-regression graph is seen on which the patient's BMD is plotted above her age. The age-regression line has a curvilinear rather than linear shape. The highest point on the line appears to be at about the age of 35, implying that peak BMD at this site is reached at about age 35. The lines paralleling the center age-regression line appear to indicate a limit of ±1 SD. Visually, then, it is clear that the patient's phalangeal BMD is both above the average peak BMD and above the value predicted for her age. The BMD is not more than 1 SD above the age-matched predicted value based on the graph. In fact, the T-score is 0.75 and the z-score is 0.84.

Figure 10-8 is a printout from a Norland Apollo™ study of the calcaneus. This is a peripheral DXA bone densitometer. According to the manufacturer, the radiation exposure to the patient during this study is less than 0.2 mrem. The calcaneus can be characterized as being an appendicular, peripheral, weight-bearing, and predominantly trabecular bone. The appearance of this printout is quite different from that seen in Fig. 10-7, but the basic information is the same. The skeletal image of the calcaneus is seen on the left, and the age-regression graph is seen on the right. The age-regression line is linear rather than curvilinear. Peak BMD appears to have been reached by the youngest age represented on the age range given on the horizontal axis of the graph, age 20. This BMD is maintained until approximately age 50, when it begins to decline. The lines paralleling the age-regression line denote a change of ±2 SDs from the age-predicted value. Once again, the patient's calcaneal BMD is plotted above her age on the graph. The actual BMD is given below the graph and is 0.646 g/cm². The percentage-comparisons and standard scores for this BMD are listed below the graph. On this graph, the green, yellow, and red color scheme is used. The cut points that determine the color changes correspond to the WHO cut points of T-scores of −1 and −2.5. A fracture risk assessment of low risk, medium risk, or high risk is given for the green, yellow, and red areas, respectively. The patient's BMD clearly falls in the green, or low-risk area. With a T-score of 0.55, the WHO diagnostic classification would be normal.

Figure 10-9 is a printout from a GE Lunar IQ™ DXA study of the proximal femur. This is a pencil-beam, DXA, central device. The image of the proximal femur is seen on the left, and the age-regression graph

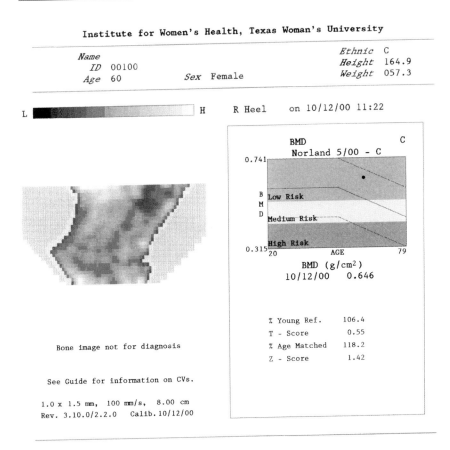

Institute for Women's Health, Texas Woman's University

Name			Ethnic	C
ID 00100			Height	164.9
Age 60		Sex Female	Weight	057.3

L [ ] H   R Heel   on 10/12/00 11:22

BMD   C
Norland 5/00 - C
0.741

B Low Risk
M
D Medium Risk

High Risk
0.315 20   AGE   79

BMD (g/cm²)
10/12/00   0.646

% Young Ref.   106.4
T - Score   0.55
% Age Matched   118.2
Z - Score   1.42

Bone image not for diagnosis

See Guide for information on CVs.

1.0 x 1.5 mm, 100 mm/s, 8.00 cm
Rev. 3.10.0/2.2.0   Calib. 10/12/00

Fig. 10-8. Norland Apollo™ DXA study of the calcaneus. Although the appearance of this report is quite different from the report in Fig. 10-7, the information that is provided is basically the same. Fracture risk categories are seen on the age-regression graph that correspond to the WHO categories of normal, osteopenia, and osteoporosis. The patient's z-score is given as 1.42. It is reasonable to assume that the limits surrounding the age-regression line indicate a change of ±2 SDs.

is seen on the right. The proximal femur itself is part of the appendicular skeleton as well as part of the central skeleton. It is clearly a weight-bearing site. The radiation exposure to the patient for this study, according to the manufacturer, is <3 mrem. Although the technologist could have chosen to emphasize any one of five different regions within the proximal femur, the total hip was chosen. The total hip itself is considered to be predominantly cortical bone, although the exact percentage of cortical bone is difficult to estimate. The choice of left hip vs right hip was

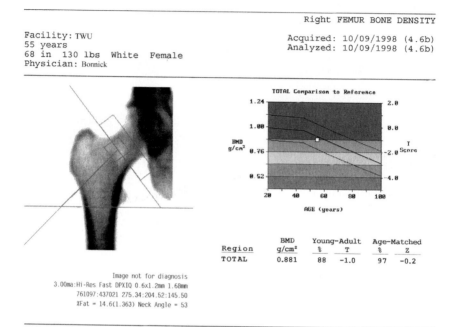

TEXAS WOMAN'S UNIVERSITY
Denton. Texas

Right FEMUR BONE DENSITY

Facility: TWU
55 years
68 in 130 lbs White Female
Physician: Bonnick

Acquired: 10/09/1998 (4.6b)
Analyzed: 10/09/1998 (4.6b)

Region	BMD g/cm²	Young-Adult % T	Age-Matched % Z
TOTAL	0.881	88 -1.0	97 -0.2

Image not for diagnosis
3.00ma:Hi-Res Fast DPXIQ 0.6x1.2mm 1.68mm
761097:437021 275.34:204.52:145.50
%Fat = 14.6(1.363) Neck Angle = 53

1 - See appendix on precision and accuracy.
  Statistically 68% of repeat scans will fall within 1 SD. (±0.02 g/cm²)
2 - USA Femur Reference Population. Young Adult Ages 20-45. See Appendices.
3 - Matched for Age, Weight(25-100kg), Ethnic.
7 - Standardized BMD for TOTAL is 831 mg/cm². See J Bone Miner Res 1994; 9:1503-1514

Fig. 10-9. GE Lunar DPX IQ™ DXA study of the proximal femur. The technologist selected the total hip ROI, and it is this value that is plotted on the age-regression graph. Note that the sBMD for the total hip BMD of 0.881 g/cm² is 831 mg/cm².

arbitrary in this case. There was no reason to suspect a difference in bone densities between the two sides since leg dominance does not appear to affect BMD in the proximal femur, as arm dominance does in the forearm.

The BMD for the total hip that was calculated from the measurement of BMC and area is given under the graph along with the percentage-comparisons and standard scores for the total hip ROI. The total hip BMD is plotted above the patient's age on the age-regression graph. On this graph, the vertical axis on the left indicates the BMD in grams/square centimeter. The vertical axis on the right indicates the T-score. The lines paralleling the age-regression line indicate a change of ±1 SD from the age-predicted value. The total hip BMD is given as 0.881 g/cm². This value is 88% of the average peak bone density of a young adult and 97%

of the value that was predicted for this 55-year-old Caucasian woman. The interpretation of these values would be that the BMD of 0.881 g/cm^2 is 12% below the average peak BMD of a young adult and 3% below the value that would otherwise be predicted for a 55-year-old Caucasian woman. It cannot be said that a 12% loss of BMD has occurred because it is not known what this patient's peak BMD was as a younger woman. Her BMD actually compares quite favorably with the BMD expected for a 55-year-old woman, but this only suggests that she does not have any secondary causes of bone loss present. The T-score of −1 indicates that the BMD of 0.881 g/cm^2 is 1 SD below the average peak bone density of the young adult. Applying the WHO criteria for diagnosis, this bone density is still normal. The z-score of −0.2 indicates that the BMD of 0.881 g/cm^2 is only 0.2 SDs below the value predicted for her age and sex. This is, again, a favorable comparison with her age-matched peers. If necessary, the BMD at the total hip of 0.881 g/cm^2 could be converted to the sBMD by using the equation found in Appendix VII. The sBMD is 831 mg/cm^2.

REFERENCES

1. Nevitt, M. C., Ross, P. D., Palermo, L., et al. (1999) Association of prevalent vertebral fractures, bone density and alendronate treatment with incident vertebral fractures: effect of number and spinal location of fractures. *Bone* **25,** 613–619.
2. Davis, J. W., Grove, J. S., Wasnich, R. D., Ross, P. D. (1999) Spatial relationships between prevalent and incident spine fractures. *Bone* **24,** 261–264.
3. Black, D. M., Arden, N. K., Palermo, L., et al. (1999) Prevalent vertebral deformities predict hip fractures and new vertebral deformities but not wrist fractures. *J. Bone Miner. Res.* **14,** 821–828.
4. Melton, L. J., Atkinson, E. J., Cooper, C., et al. (1999) Vertebral fractures predict subsequent fractures. *Osteoporos. Int.* **10,** 214–221.
5. Cummings, S. R., Black, D. M., Nevitt, M. C., et al. (1993) Bone density at various sites for prediction of hip fracture. *Lancet* **341,** 72–75.
6. Akesson, K., Gardsell, P., Sernbo, I., Johnell, O., Obrant, K. J. (1992) Earlier wrist fracture: a confounding factor in distal forearm bone screening. *Osteoporos. Int.* **2,** 201–204.
7. Marshall, D., Johnell, O., Wedel, H. (1996) Meta-analysis of how well measures of bone mineral density predict the occurrence of osteoporotic fractures. *BMJ* **312,** 1254–1259.
8. Melton, L. J., Atkinson, E. J., O'Fallon, W. M., Wahner, H. W., Riggs, B. L. (1993) Long-term fracture prediction by bone mineral assessed at different skeletal sites. *J. Bone Miner. Res.* **8,** 1227–1233.
9. Liu, G., Peacock, M., Eilam, O., Dorulla, G., Braunstein, E., Johnston, C. C. (1997) Effect of osteoarthritis in the lumbar spine and hip on bone mineral density and diagnosis of osteoporosis in elderly men and women. *Osteoporos. Int.* **7,** 564–569.

10. World Health Organization. (1994) Assessment of fracture risk and its application to screening for postmenopausal osteoporosis: report of a WHO study group. WHO Technical Report Series, WHO, Geneva.

11. Laskey, M. A., Crisp, A. J., Cole, T. J., Compston, J. E. (1992) Comparison of the effect of different reference data on Lunar DPX and Hologic QDR-1000 dual-energy X-ray absorptiometers. *Br. J. Radiol.* **65,** 1124–1129.

12. Pocock, N. A., Sambrook, P. N., Nguyen, T., Kelly, P., Freund, J., Eisman, J. A. (1992) Assessment of spinal and femoral bone density by dual X-ray absorptiometry: comparison of Lunar and Hologic instruments. *J. Bone Miner. Res.* **7,** 1081–1084.

13. Faulkner, K. G., Roberts, L. A., McClung, M. R. (1996) Discrepancies in normative data between Lunar and Hologic DXA systems. *Osteoporos. Int.* **6,** 432–436.

14. Greenspan, S. L., Maitland-Ramsey, L., Myers, E. (1996) Classification of osteoporosis in the elderly is dependent on site-specific analysis. *Calcif. Tissue Int.* **58,** 409–414.

15. Arlot, M. E., Sornay-Rendu, E., Garnero, P., Vey-Marty, B., Delinas, P. D. (1997) Apparent pre- and postmenopausal bone loss evaluated by DXA at different skeletal sites in women: the OFELY cohort. *J. Bone Miner. Res.* **12,** 683–690.

16. Varney, L. F., Parker, R. A., Vincelette, A., Greenspan, S. L. (1999) Classification of osteoporosis and osteopenia in postmenopausal women is dependent on site-specific analysis. *J. Clin. Densitom.* **2,** 275–283.

Appendix I

Contacts for Bone Densitometry Manufacturers and Organizations of Interest

MANUFACTURERS

The products listed by manufacturer refer to the products discussed in Chapter 4 and do not necessarily represent the entire line of densitometers available from the manufacturer.

Alara
2545 Barrington Court
Hayward, CA 94545-1134
Tel.: 510-723-0110
Fax: 510-723-0111
Web site: www.alara.com
E-mail: through Web site
Product: MetriScan™

CompuMed
5777 W. Century Boulevard, Suite 1285
Los Angeles, CA 90045
Tel.: 310-258-5000
Tel. (Osteo-systems): 310-258-5027
Fax: 310-645-5880
Web site: www.compumed.net or www.osteogram.com
E-mail: osteo@compumed.net
Products: Automated Osteogram®

GE Lunar
726 Heartland Trail
Madison, WI 53717-1915
Tel.: 608-828-2663
Toll-free tel.: 1-888-795-8627

Fax: 608-826-7102
Web site: www.lunarcorp.com
E-mail: info@lunarcorp.com
Technical support (through GE Cares but provided by Lunar)
    Toll-free tel.: 800-437-1171 for service or parts or
    866-225-4771 for applications
    Fax: 608-826-7107
    E-mail: Lunar.CustomerSupport@med.ge.com
Products: EXPERT®-XL, DPX-IQ™, DPX MD™, DPX MD+™,
    DPX- NT™, Prodigy™, Achilles+™, Achilles Express™,
    PIXI®

Hologic
35 Crosby Drive
Bedford, MA 01730-1401
Tel.: 781-999-7300
Toll-free tel.: 800-343-XRAY
Fax: 781-280-0669
Web site: www.hologic.com
Customer support
    Tel.: 800-321-HOLX
    E-mail: support@hologic.com
Products: QDR® 4500 A, QDR® 4500 C, QDR® 4500 SL, QDR® 4500 W,
    Delphi™, Sahara Clinical Bone Sonometer®

Norland Medical Systems
W6340 Hackbarth Road
Fort Atkinson, WI 53538
Tel.: 920-563-9504
Toll-free tel.: 800-563-9504
Fax: 920-563-8626
Customer service tel.: 800-444-8456
Technical support
    Tel.: 920-563-8456
    Fax: 920-568-4216
Web site: www.norland.com
E-mail: sales@norland.com
Products: XR-46™, Excell™, Excell™ plus, Apollo™, pDEXA®,
    McCue C.U.B.A. Clinical™

Osteometer MediTech
12515 Chadron Ave.
Hawthorne, CA 90250
Tel.: 310-978-3073
Fax: 310-676-0948
Web site: www.osteometer.com
E-mail: info@osteometer.com
Products: DexaCare™ Osteometer DTX-200, Ultrasure™ DTU-one

PronoscoAmerica
201 Penn Center Boulevard, Suite 215
Pittsburgh, PA 15235
Tel.: 877-497-6787
Fax: 412-829-5060
Web site: www.pronosco.com
E-mail: info@pronosco.com
Products: The Pronosco X-posure System™ 2.0

In Denmark
Pronosco A/S
Torsana Park, Kohavevej 5
2950-DK Vedbaek
Denmark
Tel.: 45 45 65 06 00
Fax: 45 45 65 06 10

Quidel
265 North Whisman Road
Mountain View, CA 94043
Tel.: 650-903-9400
Toll-free tel.: 800-524-6318
Fax: 650-903-9500
Web site: www.quidel.com
E-mail: through Web site
Product: QUS™-2

Schick Technologies
31-00 47th Avenue
Long Island City, New York 11101
Tel.: 718-937-5765

Toll-free tel.: 888-818-4BMD
Fax: 718-937-5962
Product support
    Toll-free tel.: 888-4-SCHICK
    Fax: 718-482-2030
Web site: www.schicktech.com
E-mail: through Web site
Product: accuDEXA™

Sunlight Medical
8 Rolling Hills, #4
Lenox, MA 01240
Tel.: 413-637-3250
Toll-free tel.: 888-460-6271
Fax: 413-637-0590
Web site: www.sunlightnet.com
E-mail: microtools-usa@msn.com
Product: Omnisense™ 7000S

In Israel
Sunlight Medical
Weizmann Science Park, Building #3
PO Box 2513
Rehovot 76100, Israel
Tel.: 972-8-930-1521
Fax: 972-8-930-1492
E-mail: info@sunlightnet.com
Web site: www.sunlightnet.com

ORGANIZATIONS OF INTEREST

American Society of Radiologic Technologists
15000 Central Avenue, S.E.
Albuquerque, NM 87123-3917
Toll-free tel.: 800-444-2778
Fax: 505-291-6072
Web site: www.asrt.org

International Society for Clinical Densitometry
2025 M Street, N.W., Suite 800
Washington, DC 20036-2422

Tel.: 202-367-1132
Fax: 202-367-2132
Web site: www.iscd.org
E-mail: iscd@dc.sba.com

National Osteoporosis Foundation
1232 22nd Street, N.W.
Washington, DC 20037-1292
Tel.: 202-223-2226
Web site: http://www.nof.org
E-mail: through Web site

Appendix II
World Health Organization Criteria for Diagnosis of Osteoporosis Based on Measurement of Bone Density[a]

Diagnosis	Bone density criteria	T-score criteria
Normal	Not more than 1 SD below the young adult peak bone density	−1 or better
Osteopenia	More than 1 but less than 2.5 SDs below the young adult peak bone density	Between −1 and −2.5
Osteoporosis	2.5 SDs or more below the young adult peak bone density	−2.5 or poorer
Severe or established osteoporosis	2.5 SDs or more below the young adult peak bone density and a fracture	−2.5 or poorer + a fracture

[a]The World Health Organization criteria were intended to be applied to measurements of bone density made only in postmenopausal Caucasian women. In the absence of other criteria, they are often applied to postmenopausal women of other races and to men of any race over the age of 50. They should not be applied to healthy premenopausal women of any race, however.

World Health Organization. (1994) Assessment of fracture risk and its application to screening for postmenopausal osteoporosis: report of a WHO study group. *WHO Technical Report Series*. WHO, Geneva.

Appendix III

National Osteoporosis Foundation Guidelines for Bone Density Measurements

Bone density measurements should be considered for the following women:

- All postmenopausal women age 65 and older
- All postmenopausal women under age 65 with one or more risk factors
- Postmenopausal women who present with fractures
- Women who have been on hormone replacement therapy or estrogen replacement therapy for prolonged periods
- Women who are considering therapy for osteoporosis if bone mineral density testing would aid decision

Risk factors to be considered in women under age 65 in supporting bone mass measurement include

- Personal history of fracture as an adult
- History of fracture in a first-degree relative
- Advanced age
- Dementia
- Poor health/frailty
- Current cigarette smoking
- Low body weight (<127 lb)
- Estrogen deficiency
  —Menopause before age 45 or bilateral oophorectomy
  —Premenopausal amenorrhea (>1 year)
- Lifelong low calcium intake
- Alcoholism
- Impaired eyesight
- Recurrent falls

- Inadequate physical activity
- History of disease associated with increased risk of osteoporosis
- History of drug use associated with increased risk of osteoporosis

National Osteoporosis Foundation. (1998) *Physician's Guide to Prevention and Treatment of Osteoporosis.* Excerpta Medica, Belle Mead, NJ.

Appendix IV
Bone Mass Measurement Act of 1997

Medicare recipients are potentially eligible for reimbursement of bone mass measurements performed in the following circumstances:

- An estrogen-deficient woman at clinical risk for osteoporosis, based on medical history and other findings
- An individual with vertebral abnormalities demonstrated by X-ray suggesting osteoporosis, osteopenia, or fracture
- An individual being monitored to assess efficacy of an FDA-approved drug therapy
- An individual receiving or expected to receive corticosteroids ≥7.5 mg of prednisone for >3 months
- An individual with primary hyperparathyroidism

Frequency Standards

At least _23_ months must have passed since the month the last measurement was performed except . . .

- For monitoring patients on long-term glucocorticoid therapy
- For allowing a confirmatory baseline measurement to permit future monitoring if the initial test was performed with a technique that is different from the proposed monitoring method

Federal Register 42 CFR Part 410; vol. 63, no. 121, June 24, 1998.

Appendix V
CPT Codes for Bone Densitometry

Technique	Skeletal site	CPT code
Dual-energy X-ray absorptiometry[a]	PA spine	76075
	Lateral spine	
	Proximal femur	
	Total body	
Dual-energy X-ray absorptiometry	Forearm	76076
	Heel	
	Phalanges	
Single-energy X-ray absorptiometry	Heel	G0130
Quantitative ultrasound	Heel	76977
Radiographic absorptiometry	Hand	76078
Computer-assisted radiogrammetry	Phalanges	76078
	Forearm	
Quantitative computed tomography[a]	PA spine	76070, G0131
	Proximal femur	
Quantitative computed tomography	Forearm	G0062
	Heel	
Single photon absorptiometry	Forearm	78350
Dual photon absorptiometry[a]	PA spine	78351
	Proximal femur	
	Total body	

[a]In the description of the code, the skeletal sites noted are characterized as axial sites, even though anatomically the proximal femur is part of the appendicular skeleton.

CPT™ codes are Level I codes developed and maintained by the American Medical Association (AMA). These are five-digit codes that are widely accepted for reporting services by health care providers. The modifier "-TC" is attached to the code to indicate billing for the technical component.

HCPCS codes, pronounced "hick-picks," are Level II codes that are developed and assigned by the Health Care Finance Administration (HCFA). They are intended to meet the needs of Medicare and Medicaid and allow coordination of government programs by providing a uniform reporting system of procedures. HCPCS codes begin with a letter and are followed by four digits. "G" codes are assigned to procedures and services that are under review for inclusion in the AMA CPT™ coding system. Once a CPT™ code is assigned, the "G" code is eliminated.

REFERENCES

AMA. HCPCS 2000. (1999) *Medicare's National Level II Codes,* 12th ed. AMA, Dover DE.

AMA. (1999) *CPT™ 2000.* AMA, Chicago, IL.

Appendix VI
DXA PA Spine Labeling Guidelines

1. Approximately 91% of women have five lumbar vertebrae.
2. The most common finding is five lumbar vertebrae with the lowest set of ribs on T12.
3. When five lumbar vertebrae are present, if the ribs are not on T12, they are usually on T11.
4. Six lumbar vertebrae are uncommon. Five lumbar vertebrae with the lowest set of ribs on T11 are more common.
5. Approximately 75% of the time, the tops of the iliac crests are in the vicinity of the L4–L5 disc space.
6. L4 is shaped like a block H or X, while L5 is shaped like a block I on its side. L1, L2, and L3 tend to be U shaped.
7. The lowest bone mineral content and bone mineral density are generally found at L1.
8. When in doubt, determine L4 and/or L5 by the shape and label from the bottom up.

Appendix VII
Conversion Formulas

PA SPINE CONVERSIONS
AMONG CENTRAL DXA DEVICES*

Hologic QDR-2000 Spine$_{BMD}$ = (0.906 × Lunar DPX-L Spine$_{BMD}$) − 0.025
Hologic QDR-2000 Spine$_{BMD}$ = (0.912 × Norland XR-26 Spine$_{BMD}$) + 0.088
Lunar DPX-L Spine$_{BMD}$ = (1.074 × Hologic QDR-2000 Spine$_{BMD}$) + 0.054
Lunar DPX-L Spine$_{BMD}$ = (0.995 × Norland XR-26 Spine$_{BMD}$) + 0.135
Norland XR-26 Spine$_{BMD}$ = (0.983 × Lunar DPX-L Spine$_{BMD}$) − 0.112
Norland XR-26 Spine$_{BMD}$ = (1.068 × Hologic QDR-2000 Spine$_{BMD}$) − 0.070

FEMORAL NECK BMD CONVERSIONS
AMONG CENTRAL DXA DEVICES*

Hologic QDR-2000 Neck$_{BMD}$ = (0.836 × Lunar DPX-L Neck$_{BMD}$) − 0.008
Hologic QDR-2000 Neck$_{BMD}$ = (0.836 × Norland XR-26 Neck$_{BMD}$) + 0.051
Lunar DPX-L Neck$_{BMD}$ = (1.013 × Hologic QDR-2000 Neck$_{BMD}$) + 0.142
Lunar DPX-L Neck$_{BMD}$ = (0.945 × Norland XR-26 Neck$_{BMD}$) + 0.115
Norland XR-26 Neck$_{BMD}$ = (0.961 × Lunar DPX-L Neck$_{BMD}$) − 0.037
Norland XR-26 Neck$_{BMD}$ = (1.030 × Hologic QDR-2000 Neck$_{BMD}$) + 0.058

*Although specific models of the central DXA devices are noted in the equations, the formulas may be used to convert BMD measured on any model for a given manufacturer to the BMD for any model of the other manufacturer. It must be recognized, however, that the error in these conversions is too great too allow serial monitoring of BMD to be done using devices from different manufacturers.

STANDARDIZED BMD (sBMD) CALCULATIONS FOR PA SPINE FOR CENTRAL DXA DEVICES*

$sBMD_{SPINE} = 1000 \ (1.0761 \times Norland \ XR\text{-}26 \ BMD_{SPINE})$
$sBMD_{SPINE} = 1000 \ (0.9522 \times Lunar \ DPX\text{-}L \ BMD_{SPINE})$
$sBMD_{SPINE} = 1000 \ (1.0755 \times Hologic \ QDR\text{-}2000 \ BMD_{SPINE})$

STANDARDIZED BMD (sBMD) CALCULATIONS FOR TOTAL HIP FOR CENTRAL DXA DEVICES*

$sBMD_{TOTAL \ HIP} = 1000 \ [(1.012 \times Norland \ XR\text{-}26 \ BMD_{TOTAL \ HIP}) + 0.026]$
$sBMD_{TOTAL \ HIP} = 1000 \ [(0.979 \times Lunar \ DPX\text{-}L \ BMD_{TOTAL \ HIP}) - 0.031]$
$sBMD_{TOTAL HIP} = 1000 \ [(1.008 \times Hologic \ QDR\text{-}2000 \ BMD_{TOTAL HIP}) + 0.006]$

*All equations are multiplied by 1000 to express the sBMD in mg/cm^2 instead of g/cm^2.

METRIC/ENGLISH CONVERSIONS FOR UNITS OF MEASURE

English to Metric	Metric to English
1 in. = 2.54 cm	1 cm = 0.39 in.
1 lb = 0.45 kg	1 kg = 2.20 lb
Degrees in F = (1.8°C) + 32	Degrees in C = (°F − 32) × 0.555
1 rad = 0.01 Gy	1 Gy = 100 rad
1 rem = 0.01 Sv	1 Sv = 100 rem

MATHEMATICAL SYMBOLS AND DESIGNATIONS OF MULTIPLES

Symbol	Designation	Factor
G	giga-	10^9
M	mega-	10^6
k	kilo-	10^3
d	deci-	10^{-1}
c	centi-	10^{-2}
m	milli-	10^{-3}
μ	micro-	10^{-6}
n	nano-	10^{-9}
p	pico-	10^{-12}

Appendix VIII

Recommended Procedures
for Short-Term Precision Studies

GENERAL PROCEDURES

1. Complete all scans within 1 month.
2. Determine precision values for each skeletal site to be used for serial measurements. The same individuals may be used for each site, however.
3. For assessing the skill level of the technologist, choose a group of individuals of normal body size in whom a normal bone density is anticipated.
4. For establishing precision values for a facility, choose a group of individuals representative of the type of patients seen at the facility.
5. Utilize an appropriate combination of number of individuals and scans per individual to give the study sufficient validity.
6. Each technologist should perform a precision study.
7. If more than 1 technologist performs bone density studies at a facility, a precision study should also be done in which all technologists participate.
8. Precision studies should be repeated if a new technologist begins work or if there is a major equipment change.

RECOMMENDED NUMBER OF INDIVIDUALS
AND NUMBER OF SCANS/INDIVIDUAL
FOR A SHORT-TERM PRECISION STUDY

No. of individuals	No. of scans/individual
10	4
15	3
30	2

CALCULATIONS

1. Calculate the average in g/cm^2 for each set of scans on an individual:

$$\overline{X}_j = \frac{\sum\limits_{j=1}^{i} X_{ij}}{n}$$

in which $\overline{X}_j$ is the average for an individual, Ms. J; $\sum\limits_{j=1}^{i}$ means to sum the first through the ith measurement; X_{ij} is each of the measured values; and n is the number of scans.

2. Calculate the SD in g/cm^2 for each set of scans on an individual:

$$SD_j = \sqrt{\frac{\sum\limits_{j=1}^{i} (X_{ij} - \overline{X})^2}{n-1}}$$

3. Calculate the percent coefficient of variation (%CV) for each individual:

$$\%CV_j = 100(SD_j/\overline{X}_j)$$

4. Calculate the average value in g/cm^2 for the entire group:

$$\overline{X}_G = \frac{\sum\limits_{m=1}^{i} \overline{X}_{im}}{m_G}$$

in which $\overline{X}_G$ is the average for the entire group, $\sum\limits_{m=1}^{i}$ means to sum the first through the ith average, $\overline{X}_{im}$ is the average for each set of measurements, and m_G is the number of individuals in the group.

5. Find the root-mean-square standard deviation (RMS-SD) in g/cm^2 for the entire group:

$$SD_{RMS} = \sqrt{\frac{\sum\limits_{m=1}^{i} (SD_{im})^2}{m_G}}$$

in which SD_{im} is the SD for each set of measurements.

6. Find the root-mean-square %CV (RMS-%CV) for the entire group:

$$\%CV_{RMS} = \left[\sqrt{\frac{\sum\limits_{m=1}^{i} (CV_{im})^2}{m_G}} \right] \times 100$$

in which CV_{im} is the CV for each set of measurements.

Appendix IX
Least Significant Change

CALCULATION OF LEAST SIGNIFICANT CHANGE (LSC)

For 1 × 1 Measurements

For a confidence level of	Multiply precision value by
99%	3.65
95%	2.77
90%	2.33
80%	1.81

For 2 × 2 Measurements

For a confidence level of	Multiply precision value by
99%	2.58
95%	1.96
90%	1.65
80%	1.28

CALCULATION OF TIME TO LSC

The time required to achieve the LSC is the time interval that should be allowed before repeating a study:

Time to LSC = LSC ÷ Anticipated Rate of Change

Appendix X
Quality Control Shewhart Rules

Rule name	Description
3 SD or 1.5% Rule	A phantom value exceeds the average ±3 SDs or 1.5%.
2 SD twice or 1.0% twice Rule	Two consecutive phantom values on the same side of the average exceed the average ±2 SDs or 1%.
Range of 4 SD or range of 2% Rule	Two consecutive phantom values differ by more than 4 SDs or 2%.
4 ± 1 SD or 4 ± 0.5% Rule	Four consecutive phantom values on the same side of the average exceed the average ±1 SD or 0.5%.
Mean × 10 Rule	Ten consecutive phantom values fall on the same side of the average, regardless of the distance from the average.

Appendix XI
Glossary of Computer Terms

Many of these terms and phrases are discussed in Chapter 5, but some are not. It is likely that the technologist will encounter all of these terms and phrases at some point in the practice of densitometry.

Applet—A very small program or application.

Application(s)—A set of instructions or a program that performs work unrelated to the actual operation of a computer itself. The programs that operate bone densitometers and analyze the data are applications. Other examples are word processors, photo editors, and spreadsheet programs.

Apps—Short for application.

ARF—An abbreviation and acronym for a common computer message indicating three possible courses of action, when an attempted action has failed. The possible actions are abort, retry or fail.

Autoexec.bat file—The file that contains instructions that must be loaded every time a computer is started. It is normally found on the C drive.

Backslash—A character on the keyboard often used in computer commands. It is important to distinguish the backslash, "\," from the forward slash, "/."

Bit—A binary digit, either 0 or 1.

Boot—To start a computer. The term comes from the old expression of "pulling yourself up by the bootstraps." In this case, the computer has to pull up, or load, its operating system in order to start and then load other programs.

Bug—An error in a computer program. The first bug was a real moth.

Bundled software—Software that is sold in conjunction with hardware.

Burn—To record a compact disk.

Bus—A mode of communication within a computer. Different modes of communication or languages are described as having different bus architectures. The bus transmits data between the input-output devices and the computer memory and central processing unit. A computer may utilize different bus architectures to communicate with various peripheral devices. Some of these different bus architectures are called ISA, PCI, VESA, USB, and FireWire. The term *bus* comes from the analogy of a bus carrying many people back and forth to different destinations. In the case of the computer, the bus carries information between the central processing unit and the various peripheral devices (like a printer or optical scanner) in both directions.

Byte—The number of bits required to indicate one character. Usually 8 bits equal 1 byte.

Card—A small circuit board that can be added to a computer by fitting or inserting it into a special slot. These circuit boards are often required in order for some peripheral devices to communicate with the computer.

CD—The abbreviation for compact disk.

CD-E—The abbreviation for compact disk-erasable. This is the same type of optical storage media as a CD-RW. CD-RW has become the preferred term.

CD-R—The abbreviation for compact disk-writable. This is a compact disk to which data or audio can be written by the user, if the computer is equipped with a CD-R drive.

CD-ROM—The abbreviation for compact disk read only memory. This is a type of optical storage media from which information can only be retrieved; information cannot be written to the CD-ROM nor can it be erased by the user.

CD-RW—The abbreviation for compact disk-rewritable. This is compact disk to which data can be written, erased, and rewritten by the user if the computer is equipped with a CD-RW drive. This type of CD is also sometimes called a CD-E, for compact disk-erasable.

Click—To briefly depress a button on the mouse.

Coaster—A compact disk that is no longer usable.

Config.sys file—A computer file that contains information on how the various devices will communicate with the computer and how computer memory is to be used. This file is normally found on the C drive.

Control-Alt-Del—A combination of keys on the keyboard that when depressed simultaneously will reboot the computer or shut down a program.

Cookie—A file from a Web site with which you have communicated that is sent to your Internet browser and stored on the hard drive that allows the Web site to identify you when you visit that site again. Some cookies may also provide additional information about you to the Web site.

CPU—The abbreviation for central processing unit. The CPU controls the operation of the computer. The microprocessor in the computer contains the CPU. The computer is often characterized by the type of CPU that it contains. For example, 80486, Pentium I, Pentium II, and Pentium III are all types of CPUs. Depending on the CPU that it contains, a computer may be called a "486" or Pentium computer.

Crash—The term indicating that the hardware has failed or an error has occurred in a program that causes the computer to become inoperable.

CRT—The abbreviation for cathode ray tube. Many computer monitors and televisions utilize CRT displays. Phosphor dots inside a glass tube are excited by an electron beam, creating an image on the screen. CRT displays are generally curved and such monitors are much heavier than liquid crystal displays.

Defrag—To use a defragmenter program.

Defragmenter—A type of utility program that organizes files on the hard drive or diskettes, making computer operations smoother.

Desktop—A term used to describe computers that are rectangular, with much greater width and depth than height, such that sitting them on a desktop is feasible. The monitor often sits on top of this computer. The term is also used to describe the opening screen of a graphic interface operating system such as Microsoft Windows®.

DIMM—The abbreviation for dual inline memory module, a type of random access memory circuit board. It is pronounced like the word, dim.

Disk, disc—Short for diskette.

Diskette—A type of magnetic data storage media. Although this term could apply to any of several different types of magnetic storage media, in common use, it refers to a 3½-in. square diskette.

Disk or disc drive—A device used to access and write data to a disk.

Double click—To briefly and in succession depress twice a button on a mouse.

Download—When a file or program is sent from a Web site to a user's computer.

DPI—The abbreviation for dots per inch. This refers to the resolution of a monitor, optical scanner, or printer. The value that is expressed is actually the dots per square inch.

DVD—The abbreviation for digital video disk. This is a type of optical storage media that can hold such large amounts of data that it is usually described in gigabytes. DVD is synonymous with DVD-ROM.

DVD-RAM—The abbreviation for digital video disk-random access memory. This is a DVD to which data can be written by the user in DVD-writable drives. This type of optical storage media is not yet in common use by personal computer users, but it offers the potential of storing gigabytes of data on one disk.

DVD-ROM—The abbreviation for digital video disk-read only memory. This is a DVD from which data can only be read; data cannot be written to this DVD by the user.

E-mail—Short for electronic mail, which are text messages sent over the Internet or other type of network.

Executable files—A file with the extension ".exe" (pronounced dot-e-x-e) or ".com" (pronounced dot-com). These files initiate programs when run by a user, rather than store data. Consequently, they are also called program files.

Extensions—Usually three or four letters that follow the period in the name of a file that indicate the type of file. For example, ".doc" is a document file. The extensions ".tif", ".pcx", and ".gif" indicate that the files are graphics files.

Firewall—Software or hardware that prevents unwanted access to computer files from an outside source.

Floppy—A type of diskette that is 3½-in. square with a hard plastic outer covering. A typical floppy disk holds approximately 1.44 MB of data.

Floppy drive—A drive that can read and write data to a floppy diskette. This drive is traditionally assigned the letter "a."

Footprint—The area or size of the space on the desktop or floor that is required by the computer.

Format—To prepare a storage media to accept data.

GB—The abbreviation for gigabyte. A measure of computer storage that contains 1 billion bytes or 1000 MB.

GUI—The abbreviation for graphic user interface. This refers to operating systems that use icons to carry out commands instead of written characters. Microsoft Windows® and Macintosh® operating systems are GUIs as opposed to DOS®, which is a character-based interface.

Hacker—An individual who accesses computer data without authorization. A computer that has been accessed illegally is said to have been "hacked."

Hard drive—A computer's internal magnetic storage media and the drive that writes data to it. It is traditionally assigned the capital letter "C" to distinguish it from drives for which there is an external access for the user, such as a floppy disk drive that is usually assigned the lowercase letter "a". The term *hard drive* is used to refer to both the drive and the storage media that the drive contains. The hard drive (or really the storage media within the hard drive) can be subdivided (or partitioned). One subdivision will retain the "C" designation, while the other subdivisions will be assigned other letters, such as "D" or "E." The lowercase letters "a" and "b" are reserved for disk drives with external user access.

Hardware—Any and all of the physical components of the computer such as the motherboard, circuitry, microprocessor, and disk drives.

Http—The abbreviation for hypertext transport protocol. This designation is normally part of the universal resource locator for a Web site or document.

Input device—Any device that allows the input of information into the computer. Examples of input devices are the keyboard, mouse, and optical scanners.

Internet—A network of smaller networks and individual computers worldwide.

ISA—The abbreviation for industry standard architecture. This is a type of bus communication.

ISP—The abbreviation for Internet service provider. This is an organization or company that provides access to the Internet by allowing the user to connect to its own computers, usually for a fee.

JPEG—The abbreviation for Joint Photographic Experts Group. This is a file extension for photographs.

KB—The abbreviation for kilobytes; 1 kilobyte = 1025 bytes.

Kbps—The abbreviation for kilobits per second. This is a unit of measure for the speed of a modem to indicate how fast data are being transmitted over a phone line; 1 Kbps = 1000 bits.

Laptop—A small computer, generally weighing under 7 lb, that opens like a notebook to reveal a screen and keyboard.

Launch—To start a program.

LCD—The abbreviation for liquid crystal display. This is a display technology used in calculators, laptop computers, and now in full-size computer monitors. LCD displays are flat and lightweight by comparison to cathode ray tube monitors.

Mac—Short for Macintosh, a type of computer operating system.

MB—The abbreviation for megabyte. This is a measure of computer storage that contains approximately 1 million bytes.

MHz—The abbreviation for megahertz. The speed of the central processing unit is measured in megahertz with 1 MHz equal to approximately 1 million cycles per second. Today's computers typically have central processing units of 500 MHz or faster.

Minitower—A tower style computer that is generally half as tall as a regular tower.

Modem—An acronym for modulator-demodulator. This device encodes data for transmission over phone lines, fiberoptic cable, or other types of communications media.

Motherboard—The main circuit board of a computer.

Mouse—An input device that allows the user to point to areas on a monitor screen and by depressing or clicking a button on the mouse initiate actions by the computer.

OCR—The abbreviation for optical character recognition. This is a type of software that allows text that has been converted to a digital image by a scanner to be converted back into text so that it can be edited on a computer.

Optical storage media—Storage media such as CD-ROM, CD-R, CD-RW, and DVD in which a laser is used to read and write data to the media.

Output device—Any device that displays the end result of the computer's calculations or actions. A monitor and printer are examples of output devices.

Parallel port—The port reserved for a cable having parallel wires, which allows data transfer at a speed of 8 bits (1 byte) at a time. This port is commonly used by printers and is designated LPT1 or LPT2. It generally has two rows of pin receptacles for a total of 25 pin receptacles to which the printer cable attaches.

PC—The abbreviation for personal computer. It also implies an IBM-compatible computer rather than a Macintosh.

PCI—The abbreviation for peripheral component interconnect, a type of bus.

Peripherals—Devices that are attached to the computer by cables. Examples are devices such as a printer, an optical scanner, a keyboard, a mouse, and a monitor.

Pixel—The smallest fragment of an image that a monitor or printer can display.

Ports—The openings or connectors on the back of the computer to which are attached the cables of the various peripheral devices, such as printers and monitors.

PS/2 port—A small round six-pin receptacle port that is designed to accept the cable from a mouse or keyboard. It was originally developed by IBM for its line of PS/2 computers but has since become the standard for other manufacturers as well.

RAM—The abbreviation and acronym for random-access memory. This is the temporary or short-term memory in the computer into which program instructions are loaded. The amount of RAM is normally measured in megabytes. Most computers today have a minimum of 64 MB of RAM.

Reboot—Restarting the computer.

Resolution—The clarity of an image on a printer or monitor. This can be measured in dots per inch or pixels.

ROM—The abbreviation and acronym for read only memory. Data can be retrieved from this memory location but cannot be written to it or erased by the user.

Scanner—An input device that converts an image or text document into a digital image that can be transferred to a computer. Text that is converted to a digital image can be changed back to text with optical character recognition software so that it can be edited like any other document.

SCSI—Pronounced "scuzzy," the abbreviation for small computer systems interface. This is a type of bus architecture. Devices that utilize SCSI to communicate with the computer are often called SCSI, or "scuzzy," devices.

SDRAM—A type of RAM circuit board.

Serial port—A port that allows data transfer at a rate of 1 bit at a time. This port is generally used for input devices such as a mouse, keyboard or bone densitometer. It generally has two rows of pins for a total of nine pins.

SIMM—The abbreviation for single inline memory module. This is a type of RAM circuit board that is found inserted into the motherboard of a computer. A computer may have more than one SIMM.

Slot(s)—A socket in a computer designed to accept add-in circuit boards. Slots are often designated by the type of communication or bus that they employ such as PCI or ISA.

Software—A set of instructions or program.

Spam—Junk e-mail. Someone who has received junk e-mail is said to have been "spammed."

Star-Dot-Star—A description of the key combination of "*.*" (the key sequence of asterisk-period-asterisk) that is used in writing the name of a file to substitute for "all files."

Super floppy—A type of diskette that contains a much greater amount of data than the traditional 1.44-MB floppy disk. Super floppies may contain more than 100 MB of data.

Tower—A computer that is much taller than it is wide such that it is generally placed on the floor, rather than on a desktop.

Upload—The opposite of download. This is when the user sends a file or program to a Web site.

UPS—The abbreviation for uninterruptible power supply. This is a device that will provide power to a computer in the event of a general power failure in order to allow the user to shut down the computer safety. The UPS generally provides 20 minutes or more of additional power, depending on the type of device purchased.

URL—The abbreviation for universal resource locator. The URL is the system used for addresses on the Internet.

USB—Universal serial bus. This was introduced in 1995 as a means of standardizing the types of connections or bus used by peripheral devices to communicate with a computer, rather than having various devices such as ISA, PCI, or VESA connections.

USB port—A port using USB.

Virus—A program that is designed to disrupt computer operation or alter or destroy data. Viruses are transmitted from computer to computer when files from an infected computer are loaded onto another computer, either by disk or by downloading from the Internet.

Web—Short for World Wide Web.

World Wide Web—The interface for the Internet.

www—The abbreviation for World Wide Web.

Zip disk—A type of magnetic storage media that holds 100 or 250 MB of data. It is approximately 3¾-in. square with a hard plastic shell.

Zip drive—A disk drive designed to read and write data to zip disks.

Zip file—A computer file that has been compressed in order to facilitate storage or transfer. It usually has the file extension ".zip". When a file is compressed, it is said to have been "zipped."

Appendix XII
Review Questions

Instructions: To obtain ASRT continuing education credit, mark your answers to the review questions on the answer sheet found in Appendix XIII. There is one single best answer to each question.

Chapter 1   An Introduction to Conventions in Densitometry

1. Which description most accurately characterizes the calcaneus?
   a. Axial, peripheral, predominantly cortical, and nonweight bearing.
   b. Appendicular, peripheral, predominantly trabecular, and weight bearing.
   c. Appendicular, central, predominantly trabecular, and weight bearing.
   d. Axial, central, predominantly cortical, and weight bearing.

2. Which of the following skeletal sites is thought to contain the highest percentage of trabecular bone?
   a. The 33% combined radial and ulnar site.
   b. The femoral neck.
   c. The 10% radial and ulnar site.
   d. The PA lumbar spine measured by dual-energy X-ray absorptiometry (DXA).

3. Which of the following statements about the standardized bone mineral density (sBMD) is *not* true?
   a. It is expressed in mg/cm^2.
   b. It reduces the differences at central sites among manufacturers to about 3%.
   c. It can be used to follow patients scanned on different manufacturers' devices over time.
   d. The formulas were based on studies of the European Spine Phantom performed on central devices from three major manufacturers.

4. The sBMD for a PA spine value of 0.932 g/cm^2 obtained using a Norland dual energy X-ray densitometer is
   a. 845 mg/cm^2.
   b. 1003 mg/cm^2.
   c. 1022 mg/cm^2.
   d. 985 mg/cm^2.

5. The bone density for three or four contiguous vertebrae is preferred to the bone density of only one or two vertebrae because
   a. There are no diseases that will affect only one vertebra.
   b. There are no reference data for BMD values from only one or two contiguous vertebrae.
   c. Accuracy and precision are superior.
   d. None of the above.

6. In densitometry, the T-score indicates the number of standard deviations above or below the predicted value for the patient's age that the patient's value actually lies:
   a. True.
   b. False.

7. The % young adult comparison can be used to indicate the amount of bone loss that a patient may have experienced:
   a. True.
   b. False

Chapter 2   Densitometry Techniques

8. The Singh Index is
   a. A type of qualitative morphometry.
   b. Based on the orderly disappearance of trabeculae in the femoral neck.
   c. Associated with fractures at values of 3 or less.
   d. All of the above.

9. The major clinical limitation of single photon absorptiometry (SPA) was
   a. Poor accuracy.
   b. Poor precision.
   c. Inability to be used to measure bone density at the spine or proximal femur.
   d. Unacceptably long scan times.

10. Compared to dual photon absorptiometry (DPA), dual energy X-ray absorptiometry (DXA) offers:
    a. Longer scan times.
    b. Equivalent image resolutions.
    c. Improved precision.
    d. Improved accuracy.

11. Which of the following statements about quantitative computed tomography (QCT) measurements of bone density in the spine is *not* true?
    a. The measurements are volumetric rather than areal measurements of bone density.
    b. Accuracy may be affected by marrow fat.
    c. Results are usually reported in g/cm^2.
    d. Trabecular bone can be isolated from cortical bone.

12. In ultrasound measurements of bone density, the speed of sound (SOS) through bone is theoretically related to both bone mass and bone quality:
    a. True.
    b. False.

13. Radiogrammetry is a technique that involves the simultaneous exposure to X ray of an aluminum wedge and the skeletal region of interest:
    a. True.
    b. False

Chapter 3   Skeletal Anatomy in Densitometry

14. Which of the following statements about the lumbar spine and PA DXA lumbar spine measurements is true?
    a. The lowest BMD is generally found at L2.
    b. Studies suggest that 83.5% of women have five lumbar vertebrae with the lowest set of ribs on T12.
    c. Osteophytes and facet sclerosis have no effect on BMD.
    d. The transverse processes of the vertebrae are included in the measurement of BMD.

15. The highest percentage of trabecular bone in the forearm is found at more proximal measurement sites:
    a. True.
    b. False.

16. The BMD in the dominant forearm is expected to be lower than in the nondominant forearm:
    a. True.
    b. False.

17. Which of the following statements is true regarding DXA proximal femur measurements?
    a. The nondominant femur should be preferentially measured.
    b. BMD is expected to be significantly higher in the dominant femur compared with the nondominant femur.
    c. Rotation of the femoral shaft has no effect on the measured BMD.
    d. Severe osteoarthritis of the hip joint can increase the measured BMD in the femoral neck.

18. Forearm sites that are named as a percentage, such as the 10% or 33% site, are named based on their location on the bone expressed as a percentage of overall radial length:
    a. True.
    b. False.

Chapter 4   Densitometry Devices Approved by the Food and Drug Administration

There are no review questions for Chapter 4.

Chapter 5   Computer Basics

19. Which of the following is not a type of magnetic storage media?
    a. Floppy diskette.
    b. Zip disk.
    c. Tape.
    d. CD.

20. The hard drive and floppy diskette drive are traditionally assigned what letters?
    a. B and c, respectively.
    b. A and d, respectively.
    c. C and a, respectively.
    d. A and b, respectively.

21. Which of the following may damage parts of a computer system?
    a. Extreme heat.
    b. High humidity.
    c. Electrical surges.
    d. All of the above.

22. Which of the following are important in preventing loss of data initially stored on the hard drive or in RAM?
    a. Regular backups to storage media.
    b. Surge protection.
    c. UPS units.
    d. All of the above.

23. The abbreviation "PC" is used to refer to computers utilizing a Macintosh operating system:
    a. True.
    b. False

Chapter 6   Precision in Bone Densitometry

24. Which combination of number of individuals and number of scans per individual is recommended for a short-term precision study?
    a. 15 individuals, 3 scans each.
    b. 10 individuals, 2 scans each.
    c. 1 individual, 10 scans.
    d. 5 individuals, 5 scans each.

25. If the precision at a skeletal site is known to be 1.2% and 1 measurement is made at baseline and again at follow-up, what percentage of increase in BMD from baseline (rounded to the nearest tenth) is required to be 80% confident that a real change in BMD has occurred?
    a. 2.2%.
    b. 3.4%.
    c. 4.5%.
    d. 5.1%.

26. By what value should the precision be multiplied to determine the least significant change at 95% confidence for one measurement at baseline and one measurement at follow-up?
    a. 1.81.
    b. 2.77.
    c. 1.96.
    d. 1.28.

27. When should a study be repeated if a change of 3% is needed to be confident that a real change has occurred and the expected rate of change is 2% per year?
    a. 1 year.
    b. 1.5 years.
    c. 2 years.
    d. 3 years.

28. If the precision of femoral neck BMD measurements is 1.4% and the measured change between two measurements is 2.8%, this change is statistically significant at the 95% confidence level:
    a. True.
    b. False.

29. A precision study should be performed
    a. At least once.
    b. When a major equipment change occurs.
    c. When a new technologist begins scanning.
    d. All of the above.

Chapter 7   Radiation Safety in X-Ray Densitometry

30. The effective radiation dose
    a. Is expressed in rads or Grays.
    b. Is the equivalent or skin dose adjusted for the sensitivity of the tissue being irradiated.
    c. Is a measure of the amount of radiation to which the specific tissue is exposed.
    d. Is greater for a PA spine DXA measurement than for a PA chest X-ray.

31. All ionizing radiation has the potential to harm living tissue:
    a. True.
    b. False.

32. If a patient is suspected of being pregnant, a DXA or QCT study
    a. May be performed anyway because the exposure is low.
    b. Should be postponed for 1 month.
    c. Should be postponed until any consideration of possible pregnancy has been eliminated.
    d. May be performed if the patient gives permission.

33. Environmental radiation typically results in an effective dose of 6 to 7 µSv/day compared to a pencil-beam DXA PA spine study that has an effective dose of 1 µSv:
    a. True.
    b. False.

34. Five rems is equivalent to how many Sieverts?
    a. 5 Sv.
    b. 1 Sv.
    c. 0.5 Sv.
    d. 0.05 Sv.

35. What is the minimum desirable distance between the technologist and X-ray tube during a DXA study?
    a. 1 ft.
    b. 3 ft.
    c. 5 ft.
    d. 10 ft.

Chapter 8   Quality Control Procedures

36. Quality control programs are less important at clinical facilities than at research facilities:
    a. True.
    b. False.

37. A quality control phantom should be measured at least three times a week and on every day a patient is studied:
    a. True.
    b. False.

38. Phantoms that mimic the size and shape of a region of the skeleton are called
    a. Linearity phantoms.
    b. Block phantoms.
    c. Hydroxyapatite phantoms.
    d. Anthropomorphic phantoms.

39. Which of the following is *not* true regarding Shewhart rules?
    a. The rules can be used in conjunction with control charts.
    b. The rules are intended to refine the identification of shifts and drifts in machine function before outright failure occurs.
    c. The rules were named for Dr. Andrew Shewhart.
    d. A violation of the rules always indicates machine malfunction.

40. A minimal quality control program should consist of recording the quality control phantom value in a table and noting whether the value falls within the established acceptable range:
    a. True.
    b. False

Chapter 9   An Overview of Osteoporosis

41. The World Health Organization criteria for the diagnosis of osteoporosis based on the measurement of bone density were intended to
    a. Establish treatment guidelines for individual patients.
    b. Establish dianostic criteria for individual patients.
    c. Result in the same diagnosis no matter what skeletal site was measured.
    d. Establish the prevalence of osteoporosis in different populations.

42. The lifetime risk of hip fracture for a Caucasian woman age 50 is estimated to be
    a. 10.0%.
    b. 15.5%.
    c. 17.5%.
    d. 19.0%.

43. The 1991 and 1993 Consensus Conference definitions of osteoporosis were notable because
    a. The definition did not refer to osteoporosis as an age-related disorder.
    b. The definition did not require the presence of a fracture for a diagnosis of osteoporosis.
    c. Osteoporosis was defined, in part, based on a measured quantity like the diseases hypertension and hypercholesterolemia.
    d. All of the above.

44. Which of the following statements about alendronate and risedronate is *not* true?
    a. Both are approved for the prevention and treatment of osteoporosis.
    b. Both are bisphosphonates.
    c. There are no significant drug interactions reported.
    d. They may be taken without regard to meals or time of day.

45. Which type of calcium supplement should be taken on an empty stomach?
    a. Calcium citrate.
    b. Calcium carbonate.
    c. Calcium phosphate.
    d. Calcium gluconate.

46. Weight-bearing exercise such as high-impact aerobics is recommended for women with low bone density:
    a. True.
    b. False.

Chapter 10   Interpretation of Bone Densitometry Data

47. Forearm sites are not generally used to monitor the effects of therapy because
    a. Precision is poor.
    b. Accuracy is poor.
    c. There is no effect of therapeutic agents on the forearm sites.
    d. The rate of change tends to be too slow.

48. In general, by how much does the risk of any type of fracture increase for a 1 standard deviation (SD) decline in BMD measured at any site?
    a. two-fold.
    b. four-fold.
    c. six-fold.
    d. eight-fold.

49. If a postmenopausal Caucasian woman has a T-score of −1 at a given skeletal site, her World Health Organization diagnostic classification would be
    a. Normal.
    b. Osteopenia.
    c. Osteoporosis.
    d. Severe osteoporosis.

50. If a healthy 30-year-old woman is found to have a PA lumbar spine T-score of −1.7, which of the following statements is true?
    a. The appropriate World Health Organization diagnostic category is normal.
    b. The appropriate World Health Organization diagnostic category is osteopenia.
    c. The appropriate World Health Organization diagnostic category is osteoporosis.
    d. World Health Organization diagnostic categories were not intended to be applied to this woman.

51. The utility of Ward's area in the proximal femur is limited in the individual because of relatively poor accuracy and precision compared to the larger regions of interest in the proximal femur:
    a. True.
    b. False.

52. A site-specific fracture risk prediction
    a. Quantifies the risk of having any type of fracture.
    b. Refers to the risk of fracture determined by measuring a specific skeletal site.
    c. Refers to the risk of fracture at a specific site, regardless of where the bone density is measured.
    d. None of the above.

INDEX

About the Authors

Sydney Lou Bonnick, MD, FACP

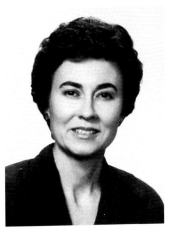

Dr. Bonnick is a native of Dallas, Texas. She is a graduate of Southern Methodist University and the University of Texas Southwestern Medical School. She is board certified in internal medicine and a fellow in the American College of Physicians. She has worked in the field of women's health with an emphasis on osteoporosis and bone densitometry for over 15 years.

Dr. Bonnick is the immediate past secretary of the International Society for Clinical Densitometry and one of the original members of the teaching faculty for the Society's physician and technologist certification programs in densitometry. She is also a member of the Scientific Advisory Board of the Bone Measurement Institute, the American Society for Bone and Mineral Research and the North American Menopause Society and a former member of the osteoporosis advisory committee for the Texas Department of Health.

She has served as a primary investigator in numerous research trials in the field of the prevention and treatment of osteoporosis and has published extensively. She is the author of two books: *The Osteoporosis Handbook* from Taylor Publishing in Dallas, Texas for patients and *Bone Densitometry in Clinical Practice* from Humana Press in Totowa, NJ for medical professionals.

Dr. Bonnick is a research professor and Medical Director for the Institute for Women's Health at Texas Woman's University in Denton, Texas.

Lori Lewis, MRT, CDT

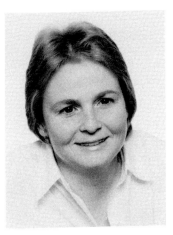

Ms. Lewis is a medical radiologic technologist and recognized by the International Society for Clinical Densitometry as a certified densitometry technologist. She is one of the original members of the technologist teaching faculty for ISCD and the 1997 winner of the ISCD technologist of the year award. She is the clinical research coordinator for Dr. Sydney Bonnick and bone density technologist at the Institute for Women's Health, Texas Woman's University in Denton, Texas. She has extensive experience in bone densitometry on all types of equipment over the last 15 years. She lives in Denton, Texas.